U0352758

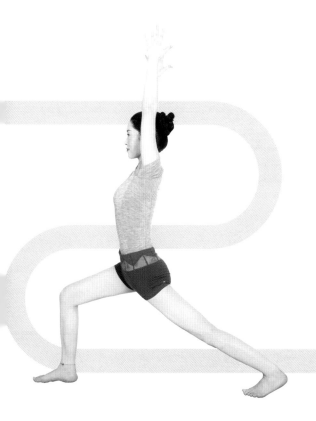

实用瑜伽英语

刘蕾 许蕾 王翔 著

四川人民出版社

前　言

　　首先，感谢公众号"瑜伽解剖学"的粉丝们，正是因为她们的热情好学、渴望知识并不断追求成为更好的自己的精神，给予我写这本书的灵感和动力。其次，感谢许蕾老师，与我一起撰写本书，并承担了大部分的修订工作。也同样感谢李丹老师的瑜伽体式演示，是她的精准示范，使得本书更具有学习价值。再次感谢李丹、许蕾、谢瑶老师在本书制作后期的详细校对，给予文章的调整建议，使得本书更加规范且方便阅读。

　　本书创作的初衷是为了给英语零基础的瑜伽人，提供一本系统学习瑜伽英语的入门书籍。从而帮助他们更容易听懂国外老师的英文瑜伽课程，阅读相关英文瑜伽书籍及网络视频，教授中/英文的瑜伽双语课程，跟讲英文的瑜伽老师或者学生实现更好的互动和沟通等。

　　本书结合实践，综合考虑瑜伽人的特点、需求及其他各方面因素，采用中英文对照的形式，尽可能多地使用简单的单词、词组和短语，少用或者尽量避开英语中的长难句来表述瑜伽教学，让零基础的、想要习得入门瑜伽英语的对象，更易学习、吸收和掌握。

当然，瑜伽领域有非常多的专业书籍，但是，至今没有一本是专门针对英语零基础的群体学习入门瑜伽英语的书籍。因此，在撰写本书的过程中，并没有现有的相关书籍作为参考，难免会存在疏漏错误及不尽完善的地方，在此抛砖引玉，希望行业领域的专家学者提出宝贵的意见，在此十分感谢！

瑜伽是一门哲学，博大精深；瑜伽也是生活的艺术，深埋智慧的宝藏，愿每一位走在路上的瑜伽人，都能满载而归。Namaste!

刘　蕾

2017 年 9 月 4 日

FOREWORD

First, I'd like to thank the fans of *Yoga Anatomy*. It is the spirit they show when they are eager for knowledge in pursuit of the optimal level of oneself that has been pushing me forward; next, I will appreciate my junior female schoolmate Xu Lei for co-writing the book with me, who undertook most of the revision work. I also want to thank my friend Li Dan who demonstrated the yoga asana precisely, which makes the book more accessible. Finally, I would like to thank Li Dan, Xu Lei, and Xie Yao again for their proofreading and suggestions in the later stage of writing the book, for it to be more standardized and easier to read.

The original intention of this book is to provide a systematic reference of yoga English for the zero-based yogis. It will help them understand foreign teachers'yoga courses better, read yoga books in English, watch online yoga videos without Chinese subtitles, teach yoga bilingual courses, and communicate with English-speaking yoga teachers or students better, etc..

Combined with practice and considering yogis' characteristics, needs and other factors, the whole book is written in both Chinese and English. In addition, this book tries to use simple words and phrases to express yoga teaching, and to avoid adopting long and complicated sentences in English, so that zero-based yoga learners can feel easier to learn, master and absorb the content.

For now, there are a lot of professional books about yoga, but so far there is no one book that specializes in yoga English for zero-based learners. Therefore, in the process of writing this book, there is no existing related book on yoga English as a reference. It is inevitable that there will be omissions and incompleteness, and I hope that the experts and scholars in the professional field can put forward valuable suggestions. I would appreciate it very much.

Yoga is a philosophy; it is profound. Yoga is the art of life; it is full of wisdom. I wish every yogi who walks on the road can come back with fruitful results. Namaste!

Liu Lei

Sept.4, 2017

目　录

CONTENTS

第 1 章　瑜伽英语常用名词
Chapter 1　Nouns in Yoga English

1. 身体部位常用名词 Nouns about our body

（1）头部 Head

前额 forehead	眉毛 brow	眼睛 eye
脸 face	鼻子 nose	嘴巴 mouth
舌头 tongue	耳朵 ear	下巴 chin
头发 hair	头皮 scalp	

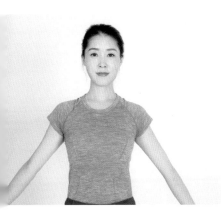
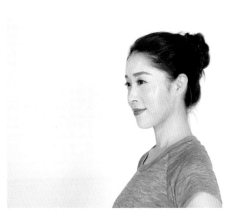

（2）躯干 Body

颈部 neck　　　　锁骨 collarbone　　　肩膀 shoulder

胸部 chest　　　　肋骨 rib　　　　　　背部 back

腹部 belly/abdomen　　髋部 hip　　　　髋关节 hip joint

臀部 buttock　　　脊柱 spine　　　　　骶骨 sacrum

耻骨 pubis　　　　骨盆 pelvis　　　　腰部 waist

髂骨 ilium　　　　坐骨 ischium

肩胛骨 shoulder blade/scapula

胸骨 breastbone/sternum

胸椎 thoracic vertebrae

腰椎 lumbar vertebrae

尾骨 tailbone/coccyx

颈椎 cervical vertebrae

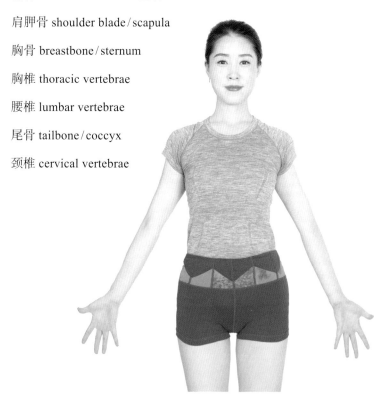

1

（3）上肢 Upper limbs

手臂 arm

前臂 forearm

大臂 upper arm

小臂 lower arm

腋窝 armpit

手肘 elbow

肘关节 elbow joint

手腕 wrist

手 hand

手掌 palm

手背 back of the hand

手指 finger

大拇指 thumb

食指 index finger

中指 middle finger

无名指 ring finger

小指 little finger

指尖 finger tips

指根 finger roots

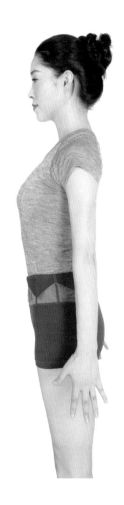

（4）下肢 Lower limbs

大腿 upper leg/thigh　　　膝盖 knee　　　膝关节 knee joint

膝盖（髌）骨 knee cap/patella　　　脚踝 ankle

腘窝（膝盖窝）popliteal fossa (space)　　　踝关节 ankle joint

大脚球 the big ball of foot

足弓 arch

小腿 lower leg/shank

脚掌 sole

足跟 heel

脚 foot

脚背 instep

脚趾 toe

大脚趾 big toe

二脚趾 index toe

三脚趾 middle toe

四脚趾 forth toe

小脚趾 little toe

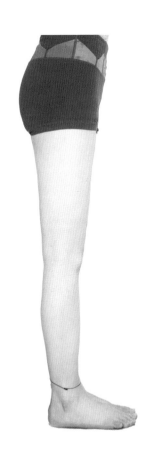

1

（5）肌肉 Muscle

三角肌 deltoid

肱二头肌 biceps brachii

肱三头肌 triceps brachii

斜方肌 trapezius

背阔肌 latissimus dorsi

胸大肌 pectoralis major

胸小肌 pectoralis minor

前锯肌 serratus anterior

横膈膜 diaphragm

腰大肌 psoas major

腰方肌 quadratus lumborum

腹直肌 rectus abdominis

腹横肌 transversus abdominis

腹内斜肌 internal oblique

腹外斜肌 external oblique

臀大肌 gluteus maximus

臀中肌 gluteus medius

臀小肌 gluteus minimus

梨状肌 piriformis

腘绳肌 hamstring

股四头肌 quadriceps

腓肠肌 gastrocnemius

（6）其他 Others

胃 stomach

肺 lung

心脏 heart

肾脏 kidney

子宫 uterus

膀胱 bladder

会阴 perineum

腹股沟 groin

韧带 ligament

2. 瑜伽辅具常用名词 Nouns about yoga props

辅具 prop　　　　　辅助绳 rope　　　凳子 stool

椅子 chair　　　　　毛毯 blanket　　　瑜伽球 yoga ball

瑜伽垫 yoga mat　　瑜伽砖 yoga block

泡沫滚轴 foam roller　瑜伽抱枕 yoga bolster

瑜伽轮 yoga wheel　瑜伽枕 yoga pillow

瑜伽伸展带 yoga belt / strap

圆形木砖 round wooden block

瑜伽弹力带 yoga fitness resistance band / elastic latex belt

1

3. 瑜伽教室常用名词 Nouns about yoga classroom

瑜伽工作室 yoga studio　　　　瑜伽教室 yoga class

瑜伽音乐 yoga music　　　　　桌子 desk

地板 floor　　　　　　　　　天花板 ceiling

窗户 window　　　　　　　　墙 wall

门 door　　　　　　　　　　角落 corner

灯 light　　　　　　　　　　镜子 mirror

讲台 platform

4. 瑜伽教学常用名词 Nouns about yoga teaching

书 book	组 group	序列 sequence
主题 theme	疼痛 pain	学校 / 流派 school
练习 practice	治疗 therapy	健康 health
方法 method	讲座 lecture	示范 demonstration
调整 alignment	问题 problem	

时间 time	小时 hour	分钟 minute
秒钟 second	天 day	周 week
月 month	年 year	

核心 core	力量 strength	柔韧性 flexibility
平衡性 balance	速度 speed	耐力 stamina
体能 physical ability	运动 movement	

态度 attitude	意识 awareness	冥想 meditation
热情 passion	状态 condition	简单 simplicity
平静 peace	感觉 feeling	情绪 emotion
稳定 stability	不稳定 instability	控制 control
压力 pressure / stress	努力 effort	紧张 tension

第 2 章　瑜伽体式常用引导动词及动词短语
Chapter 2　Verbs and Verb Phrases in Yoga Poses

站立 stand　　　　坐立 sit　　　　跪立 kneel

仰卧 lie face up/lie flat on the back/lie on the back/lie down on the
　　back

俯卧 lie face down/lie flat on the stomach/lie on the abdomen/
　　lie down on the abdomen

上提 lift/raise/push up　　　　　　下沉 drop/lower

收紧 tighten/contract/flex　　　　　放松 relax

打开 open　　　　转动 roll/rotate/turn　扭转 twist

移动 move　　　　倾斜 lean　　　　放置 put/land/place

支撑 support/prop　保持 hold/keep/remain/maintain

拉伸 stretch　　　延伸 extend/elongate　加强 strengthen

伸直 straighten　　垂直 be perpendicular to

折叠 fold　　　　弯曲 bend　　　　平行 parallel

松开 release　　　抓住 grip/grasp/catch/hold

交叉 cross　　　　交换 switch　　　交扣 interlock

交握 clasp　　　　还原 return　　　转移 transfer

平衡 balance　　　　跳跃 jump　　　　分开 spread

开始 start/begin　　　结束 end　　　　吸气 inhale/breathe in

呼气 exhale/breathe out

第 3 章　瑜伽体式方位引导介词（短语）和副词
Chapter 3　Prepositions and Adverbs in Yoga Poses

向上 up / upward

向下 down / downward

向前 front / forward

向后 back / backward

左边 left

右边 right

上面 on

下面 under

前面 in front of

后面 behind

内侧 inner side / inside

外侧 outer side / outside

两侧 both sides of

两者之间 between

三者（及以上）之间 among

在……中间 in the middle of

在……中心 in the center of

……度 at an angle of ... degree

第4章　瑜伽体式练习中常用口令短语
Chapter 4　Instruction Phrases Used in Yoga Practice

双肩放松下沉

relax and lower your shoulders

双手侧平举

reach out your hands to shoulder level

双脚并拢站立

stand with feet together

延展脊柱

elongate your spine

大腿收紧

tighten your thighs

膝盖骨上提

lift your knee caps

山式开始

start in mountain pose

身体与地面平行

keep your body parallel to the floor

双脚站立，打开……距离

stand with feet wide about ... apart

屈膝 90 度

bend knees to 90 degrees

屈前膝

bend the front knee

屈肘

bend elbows

肩胛骨下沉

shoulder blades down

保持双腿伸直

keep both legs straight

将脚放在大腿内侧

put your foot onto inner side of the thigh

仰卧屈双膝

lie face up with knees bent

双脚平放在地面

feet flat on the floor

双臂在身体两侧

arms at sides

双脚平行且与髋同宽

keep feet parallel and hip-width apart

抬髋部向上离开地面

lift the hips off the floor

掌心朝上

palms face up

闭上眼睛放松

close eyes and relax

转胸腔向上

turn your chest up

胸腔打开

open the chest

胸腔上提展开

lift and spread your chest

跪立，双腿打开且与髋同宽

kneel with legs hip-width apart

双腿伸直坐立

sit and straighten legs out in front of you

屈双膝坐立

sit with knees bent

手臂向前伸直

stretch arms forward

肩膀后展

push your shoulders back

均匀地呼吸

breathe evenly

放松右侧髋关节

relax the right hip joint

身体不要向后倾斜

do not allow your torso to lean back

放松颈部的肌肉

relax your neck muscles

加强左腿的伸展

intensify the stretch of your left leg

收紧臀部，尾骨向下

tighten your buttocks and pull your tailbone down

双脚分开约 1.2 米的距离

spread your feet about 1.2 meters apart

双手平放于地面

keep your palms flat on the floor

腹部内收

draw the abdomen / belly in

肩胛骨相互靠拢

draw your shoulder blades toward each other

双脚外侧平行

keep the outer edges of your feet parallel to each other

大腿向下压

press your thighs down

脚趾分开

spread your toes

手臂延展远离身体

lengthen your arms away from the body

肩膀在髋部的正上方

shoulders aligned over hips

后脚向外打开 90 度

back foot angled out about 90 degrees

膝盖在脚踝的正上方

knees directly over ankles

前脚后跟与后脚足弓在一条直线上

front heel aligned with arch of back foot

保持核心收紧有力

keep your core tight and strong

侧腰延展

keep your sides of torso lengthened

手腕在肩膀的正下方

wrists right under shoulders

颈部、躯干和双腿在一条直线上

keep your neck, torso and legs in a line

眼睛看向前方

gaze forward / look ahead

肩膀远离耳朵

keep your shoulders away from ears

髋部远离地面

lift your hips away from floor

保持中立位

keep in the neutral position

第 5 章　瑜伽练习的益处、禁忌等常用名词及短语

Chapter 5　Nouns and Phrases About Benefits, Taboos and Cautions of Yoga Poses

1. 瑜伽练习的益处常用短语 Benefits of yoga practice

拉伸双肩和颈部

stretch the shoulders and neck

加强手臂、双腿和脊柱

strengthen arms, legs and spine

刺激腹部器官

stimulate abdominal organs

按摩腹部器官

massage abdominal organs

缓解疲劳和焦虑

reduce fatigue and anxiety

缓解背部 / 颈部 / 髋部疼痛

relieve back / neck / hip pain

缓解压力

relieve stress / pressure

减轻抑郁情绪

mild depression

冷静大脑

calm the brain

治疗哮喘和失眠

therapeutic value for asthma and insomnia

改善背部 / 脊柱 / 髋部的柔韧性

improve back / spine / hip flexibility

改善睡眠质量

improve sleep quality

纠正不良体姿

correct bad posture

促进消化

improve digestion

促进血液循环

improve the blood circulation

加强核心力量

strong the body's core

打开肩部 / 髋部

open shoulder / hip

减重

lose weight

降低高血压

lower high blood pressure

缓解坐骨神经痛

ease the sciatica

防止受伤

avoid injury

缓解肌肉紧张

minimize muscle tension

抵抗衰老

reverse aging

缓解关节炎

alleviate arthritis

提高专注力和注意力

boost focus and concentration

促进新陈代谢

invigorate metabolism

抵制骨质疏松

counteract osteoporosis

加深排毒

assist detox

增强免疫系统

strengthen immune system

滋养心灵

nourish the soul

增强耐力

enhance endurance

保持年轻

stay young

2. 瑜伽练习的禁忌或注意事项常用语 Taboos and cautions of yoga practice

练习瑜伽前避免吃得过多。

Avoid eating too much before yoga practice.

最好空腹练习。

Try not to eat anything before practicing yoga.

不要屏息。

Do not hold your breath.

不要用嘴呼吸。

Do not breathe through your mouth.

瑜伽练习后过 15 分钟再淋浴。

Wait 15 minutes and bath after yoga practice.

不要攀比。

Do not compare with others.

最佳练习时间是黎明或傍晚。

The best time of practicing is at dawn or at dusk.

练习地点保持空气流通 。

Keep air circulation at the practicing place.

禁止噪音。

No noise.

5

大脑保持警醒。

Keep your brain sober.

身体放松，不要有压力。

Relax your body without pressure.

经期尽量避免练习。

Avoid practicing during your period.

产后第一个月不应练习任何体式。

Avoid practicing any yoga asana after a month postpartum.

当你感觉头脑清醒充满活力再开始体式练习。

Practise asana when you feel fresh and energetic.

不要以后弯体式开始你的练习。

Do not begin your session with backbend asana.

练习不同类型的体式。

Practise different types of asana.

保持精力集中。

Concentrate completely.

3. 其他常用名词及短语 Other nouns and phrases of yoga practice

心脏病 heart disease　　　　头痛 headache

月经 menstruation　　　　　生理期 on one's period

怀孕 pregnancy　　　　　　腹泻 diarrh(o)ea

哮喘 asthma　　　　　　　偏头疼 migraine

高 / 低血压 high / low blood pressure

鼠标手（腕管综合征）carpal tunnel syndrome

肩部僵硬（冻肩）frozen shoulder

失眠 insomnia　　　　　　圆肩 rounded shoulders

平脊 flat back　　　　　　驼背 hunchback

异常凹背 swayback　　　　脊柱前凸 lordosis

脊柱侧弯 scoliosis　　　　腹部肌肉弱 weak abdomen

腰椎间盘突出 lumbar intervertebral disc herniation

髂腰肌紧张 tight iliopsoas　臀大肌弱 weak gluteus maximus

膝盖超伸 knees hyper-extended

O 型腿（弓形腿）bow legs

5

X 型腿（膝外翻）knock knees   扁平足 flat feet

骨盆前倾 anterior pelvis tilt

骨盆后倾 posterior pelvis tilt

头前倾 forward head

上交叉综合征 upper crossed syndrome

下交叉综合征 lower crossed syndrome

第6章 31个常用瑜伽基础体式引导口令
Chapter 6　Instruction of 31 Classic Yoga Poses

---

1. 站姿体式 Standing poses

（1）山式 Mountain pose / Tadasana

双脚并拢。

Feet together.

脚内侧和外侧均衡地向下压。

Press the inner and outer side of your feet evenly into the floor.

大腿肌肉收紧，髌骨上提。

Tighten your thigh muscles. Pull your knee caps upward.

大腿前侧向后推，双腿垂直于地面，身体重心均匀分布在双脚上。

Turn the front of your thighs backward. Legs are perpendicular to the floor. Distribute your weight equally on the feet.

尾骨顺向地面。

Lengthen your tailbone toward the floor.

伸直脊柱，胸腔上提打开。

Spine straight, lift and open your chest.

双肩下沉。

Lower the shoulders down.

手臂沿身体两侧伸直向下。

Extend your arms along the sides of your body.

保持颈部、头部伸直，目视前方。

Keep your head and neck upright. Look straight ahead.

保持自然地呼吸。

Breathe normally and naturally.

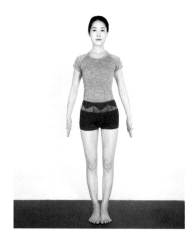
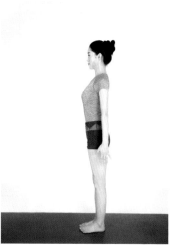

（2）幻椅式 Chair pose / Utkatasana

山式站立。

Stand in mountain pose.

吸气，双手经体前向上举过头顶，掌心相对。

Inhale, and raise your arms overhead, with your palms facing each other.

大臂靠近耳朵，手肘伸直。

Keep your upper arms close to your ears, elbows straight.

呼气，臀部向后下坐 。

Exhale; sit your buttocks down.

感觉自己坐在一把椅子上。

Feel like sitting in a chair.

重心均匀分布在双脚上。

Distribute your weight evenly on your feet.

大腿肌肉收紧，腹股沟向后，背部伸展。

Tighten your thigh muscles. Groin backward. Stretch your back.

6

紧收肋骨，胸腔上提。

Tighten your ribs. Lift your chest up.

手臂与身体成一条直线；双肩下沉。

Keep your arms and torso in a line. Release shoulders down.

保持 3~5 次缓慢的呼吸。

Hold this pose for three to five slow breaths.

吸气，还原为山式。

Inhale, and return to mountain pose.

（3）鸟王（鹰）式 Eagle pose / Garudasana

山式站立，屈双膝。

Stand in mountain pose. Bend your knees.

身体重心移向右腿。

Transfer your weight to the right leg.

抬左腿向上，缠绕右大腿，左脚缠绕在右腿肚后侧。

Lift the left leg up, and twist your right thigh, then hook your left foot behind the lower right calf.

双手侧平举。

Reach your arms out to your sides to a T shape.

右手臂在上，左手臂在下，相互缠绕，掌心相对。

Cross your left arm under the right. Wind the right forearm around the left. Bring your palms together.

大臂平行于地面，小臂垂直于地面。

Upper arms are parallel to the floor; lower arms are perpendicular to the floor.

支撑腿的膝盖朝向脚尖，双腿收紧。

Keep your knee of the standing leg toward the tiptoes. Tighten your legs.

髋部朝前，延展背部向上。

Keep your hips forward. Stretch your back up.

保持 3~5 次呼吸。

Keep three to five breaths.

吸气，解开双腿双手。

Inhale, and unwind legs and hands.

还原为山式。换另一侧练习。

Return to mountain pose. Repeat on the other side.

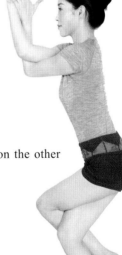

6

（4）树式 Tree pose / Vrksasana

山式站立。

Stand in mountain pose.

左脚着地，左膝向外侧打开。

Put the toes of your left foot on the floor. Open your left knee out to the side.

抬左脚，将脚掌放在右大腿内侧。

Lift your left foot off the floor. Place the sole against the inner right thigh.

左脚脚跟靠近会阴，脚尖指向正下方。

Draw the left heel close to your perineum, toes pointing toward the floor.

右脚内侧踩实，右腿垂直于地面。

Press the inner side of right foot into the floor. Keep your right leg perpendicular to the floor.

双腿肌肉收紧，左脚与右大腿互抵用力。

Tighten muscles of your legs. Press your left foot into your right thigh, which back into your left foot with equal pressure.

髋部中正，保持身体重心的稳定。

Keep your hips in the neutral position. Keep your weight stable.

双手臂向上举过头顶，双手与肩同宽，掌心相对。

Raise your hands overhead. Open your arms shoulder-width apart, palms facing each other.

双肩放松，眼睛平视前方一个固定的点。

Shoulders relaxed, gaze at a fixed point in front of you.

保持 3~5 次呼吸，呼气，左脚落地，放下手臂。

Keep three to five breaths. Exhale, and lower your left foot to the floor. Release your arms to your sides.

换另一侧练习。

Repeat on the other side.

（5）三角伸展式 Triangle pose/Trikonasana

山式站立，双腿分开约 1.2 米宽。

Stand in mountain pose, with your legs about 1.2 meters apart.

保持双脚外沿平行；脚趾朝前，双手侧平举。

Keep the outer edges of your feet parallel. Toes forward, reach arms out to your sides to a T shape.

6

转右脚 90 度，左脚微内扣。

Turn your right foot out 90 degrees to the right. Turn your left foot slightly to the right.

右脚脚跟与左脚足弓在一条直线上。

Right heel and left arch should be in a line.

右大腿肌肉收紧外旋；右膝盖与第二、三根脚趾在一条直线上。

Rotate your right thigh muscles outward. Keep your right knee in a line with the index toe and middle toe of right foot.

呼气，伸展躯干，身体向右、向下弯曲。

Exhale and stretch your torso. Bend your torso down to the right.

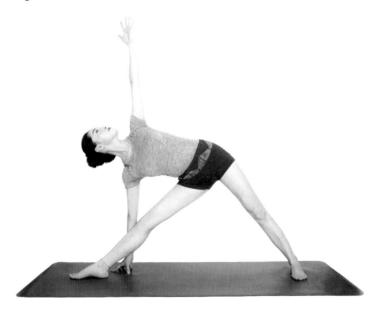

拉伸时尽量保持两侧腰等长。

Keep both sides of your torso the same stretch as possible.

右手放在小腿胫骨的外侧或者瑜伽垫上。

Put your right hand on the outer side of your shin or on the mat.

左手指向天花板。

Left hand pointing toward the ceiling.

转腹部及胸腔向前。

Turn your abdomen and chest forward.

转头，眼睛看向天花板的方向。

Turn your head and gaze toward the ceiling.

保持 3~5 次呼吸，吸气，蹬后腿，立直上半身。

Keep three to five breaths. Inhale and straighten your back leg.
Keep your upper body straight.

转右脚朝前；换另一侧练习。

Turn your right foot forward. Repeat on the other side.

6

（6）战士二式 Warrior pose II / Virabhadrasana II

山式站立，双腿分开大于 1.2 米。

Stand in mountain pose with your legs more than 1.2 meters apart.

保持双脚外沿平行；脚趾朝前，双手侧平举。

Keep the outer edges of your feet parallel. Toes forward, reach
your arms out to your sides to shoulder level.

右脚向外转90度，左脚微内扣，左足弓与右脚跟在一条直线上。右脚脚尖正对右侧方向。

Turn your right foot out to the right in 90 degrees. Keep left foot to the right slightly. Align the left arch with the right heel, toes of your right foot pointing toward the right.

吸气，脊柱延伸；呼气，蹬左腿，屈右膝，使小腿与地面垂直；大小腿互相成90度。

Inhale, spine straight. Exhale, stretch your left leg. Bend your right knee. Make the shin perpendicular to the floor. Keep your upper right leg and your lower right leg at an angle of 90 degrees.

右膝对准右脚趾尖的方向，向右转头，眼睛看向右手指尖。

Keep your right knee cap in line with your right toes. Turn the head to the right. Look over the fingers of right hand.

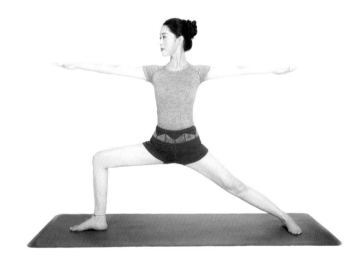

骨盆保持中正，脊柱向上伸展。

Keep your pelvis in the neutral position, spine straight.

保持这个姿势 3~5 次呼吸，换另一侧练习。

Stay in the pose for three to five breaths.Repeat on the other side.

（7）战士一式 Warrior pose I/ Virabhadrasana I

山式站立，双脚分开约 1.2 米宽，双手扶髋。

Stand in mountain pose with your legs about 1.2m apart. Place your hands on hips.

转右脚朝向正右方。左脚跟抬高，同时将髋部也转向右侧，两脚内侧在一条直线上。

Turn your right foot in 90 degrees to the right. Lift your left heel and rotate your hips to the right. Keep the inner sides of your feet in a line.

吸气，双臂从体前上举过头顶。

Inhale, and raise your arms overhead in front of your body.

呼气，蹬直左腿；屈右膝，右小腿垂直地面，膝盖对准脚尖。

Exhale, and straighten your left leg. Bend your right knee. The right shin should be perpendicular to the floor. Align right knee with your tiptoes.

左腿伸直，左脚跟蹬向地面，骨盆中正。

Keep your left leg straight. Press the left heel firmly into the floor. Keep the pelvis in a neutral position.

脊柱向上伸展，展开胸腔和腋窝，大臂尽量靠近耳朵，手肘伸直，双肩下沉。

Lengthen the spine. Expand your chest and armpits. Make your upper arms close to your ears. Straighten elbows and lower your shoulders down.

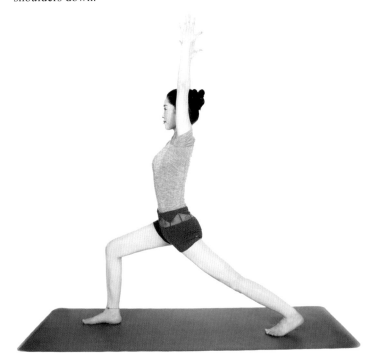

吸气，伸直双腿，转脚朝前，换至对侧练习。

Inhale, straighten your legs and turn the feet forward. Repeat on the other side.

（8）加强侧伸展式 Sideways Extension / Parsvottanasana

山式站立，双脚分开不超过 1.2 米宽，双手扶髋。

Stand in mountain pose with your legs less than 1.2m apart. Place your hands on hips.

转左脚向左 90 度，右脚跟抬高将髋部转向正左侧，右脚跟在地面踩实。

Turn your left foot to the left in 90 degrees. Lift your right heel and rotate your hips to the left. Press your right heel firmly on the floor.

吸气，展开胸腔，手肘后展。

Inhale, and expand your chest with elbows backward.

呼气，从腹股沟起向前、向下弯曲躯干。双手落于肩膀正下方，眼睛看向前方。

Exhale, and bend your torso forward and down from the groin. Hands are under your shoulders. Gaze forward.

6

两脚内侧踩实，双腿收紧，右腿向后伸直，髋部中正。

Press the inner edges of your feet firmly on the floor. Tighten your legs and straighten your right leg. Keep your hips in a neutral position.

胸骨向前伸展，背部展平，双肩后展。

Lift your sternum forward. Keep your back flat and expand shoulders backward.

吸气，手扶髋直立起身，转脚朝前，换至对侧练习。

Inhale, rouse yourself, with hands on hips. Turn your feet forward. Repeat the pose on the other side.

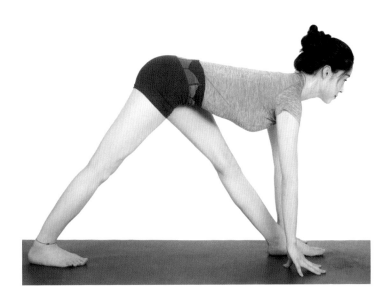

2. 坐姿体式 Sitting poses

（9）手杖式 Staff pose / Dandasana

坐立在垫面上，拨动臀部向后向外，让坐骨坐实地面。

Sit on the mat. Draw your buttocks backward and outward. Press your ischium into the floor.

双脚及双腿并拢，脚趾指向天空。

Keep your feet and legs together with your toes pointing toward the sky.

双手放在臀部两侧，指尖朝前。

Put your hands by the sides of buttocks, with your fingertips pointing forward.

大腿肌肉收紧，腿后侧压向地面。

Tighten your thigh muscles and press the back of your legs into the floor.

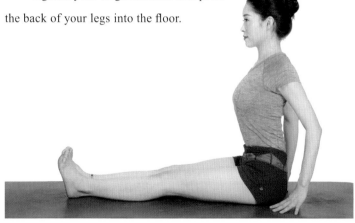

6

骶骨上提，胸腔展开，收肋骨。

Lift your sacrum and open your chest. Ribs in.

展开肩膀并下沉，头在脊柱的延长线上。

Open and lower your shoulders. The head is on the extension line of your spine.

保持顺畅地呼吸。

Breathe smoothly.

（10）简易坐式 Easy pose / Sukhasana

手杖式坐立，屈双膝。

Sit in staff pose, and bend your knees.

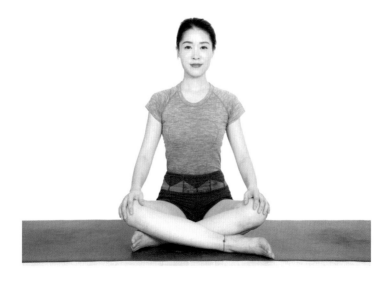

让两小腿在中段处相交叉，双膝落在双脚的正上方。

Cross your legs from the middle of shanks, with the knees directly over your feet.

双手放在膝盖上方，掌心朝下。

Rest your hands over your knees, palms facing down.

吸气，脊柱向上立直；呼气，放松双肩。

Inhale, spine extended upward. Exhale, shoulders relaxed.

颈部后侧伸展向上，目视前方，让你的意念集中。

Extend the back of your neck upward. Gaze forward and concentrate your mind.

停留 3~5 次呼吸，解开双腿，换另一侧练习。

Stay in this pose for three to five breaths. Uncross your legs and repeat on the other side.

（11）坐角式 Seated wide-angle pose / Upavisata Konasana

手杖式坐立，双腿尽量向外打开。

Sit in staff pose, and spread your legs apart as far as possible.

膝盖和脚趾指向天花板。

Knees and toes point toward the ceiling.

大腿肌肉收紧压向垫面，两脚内侧向前推。

Tighten your thigh muscles and press them into the floor. Push the inner side of your feet forward.

6

吸气，双手侧平举，脊柱向上立直。

Inhale, and reach out your arms to a T shape. Keep your spine erect.

呼气，身体向前、向下弯曲。

Exhale, and fold your upper body forward and down.

双手中间三指抓大脚趾，亦可用双手握住双脚脚掌。

Catch your big toes with your middle three fingers, or you can hold your soles with your hands.

骶骨向前，胸腔展开，同时延展背部，肩膀下沉远离耳朵。

Draw your sacrum forward. Open your chest and extend your back downward. Shoulders down away from your ears

保持这个体式 3~5 次呼吸，吸气，还原为手杖式。

Stay in this pose for three to five breaths. Inhale and return to staff pose.

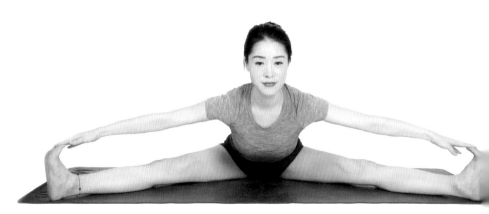

（12）束角式 Bound angel pose / Baddha Konasana

手杖式坐立，弯曲双膝。

Sit in staff pose, and bend your knees.

两脚掌互抵，将脚跟尽量靠近会阴。

Soles of your feet are set against each other. Draw your heels close toward your perineum.

双手分别抓住两个大脚趾，双膝向下靠近地面。

Hold your big toes with both hands. Press your knees to the floor.

骶骨上提，脊柱立直，展开胸腔及肩膀，目视前方。

Lift your sacrum up. Spine straight, stretch out your chest and shoulders. Gaze forward.

6

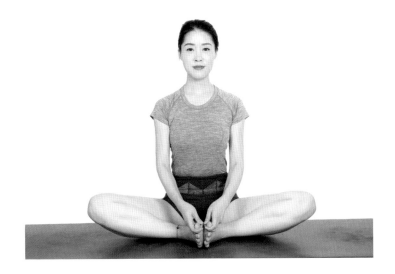

保持这个姿势 3~5 次呼吸，还原为手杖式。

Stay in this pose for three to five breaths and return to staff pose.

（13）单腿头碰膝式 Head-on-knee pose / Janu Sirsasana

手杖式坐立，屈左膝。

Sit in staff pose. Bend your left knee.

左脚掌紧紧贴放在右大腿根部，弯曲的膝盖沉向垫面。

Put your left sole on the inside of your right thigh. Make sure that your bent knee is pressed firmly down to the mat.

吸气，双手上举过头顶，大臂贴靠耳朵。

Inhale, and lift arms up above your head, with upper arms close to your ears.

呼气，从腹股沟起，身体向前、向下弯曲。

Exhale, and bend your body forward and down from the groin.

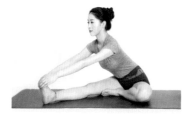 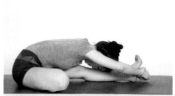

双手抓住左前脚掌，拉长脊柱，延展背部。

Hold the front of your left sole with your hands. Stretch the spine and elongate your back.

保持 3~5 次呼吸，还原为手杖式。

Keep three to five breaths and return to staff pose.

(14) 牛面式 Cow head pose / Gomukhasana

手杖式坐立，屈双膝。

Sit in staff pose and bend your knees.

将右脚从左膝下方穿过，脚背放于左臀外侧。

Cross the right foot under your left knee. Place your right instep by the outer side of your left buttock.

将左脚放于右臀外侧，双膝交叠，坐骨均匀地坐实地面。

Place your left foot by the outer side of your right buttock. Cross your knees. Press your ischium into the ground evenly.

双手侧平举，左臂向上，弯曲左肘，左手掌放于上背部。

Reach out your arms to your sides to a T shape. Bring your left arm up to the sky. Bend the left elbow so the left palm rests on the upper back.

6

右臂向后、向下，弯曲右肘，左右手互拉。

Bring the right arm back and down. Bend your right elbow. Your left hand and right hand should be able to hold each other.

脊柱立直，双肩展开，两手肘上下对抗，并向中线靠拢。

Keep spine straight, stretch out your shoulders. Elbows confront each other to close the centre line of spine.

保持这个姿势 3~5 次呼吸，然后换另一侧练习。

Hold the pose for three to five breaths and then switch sides.

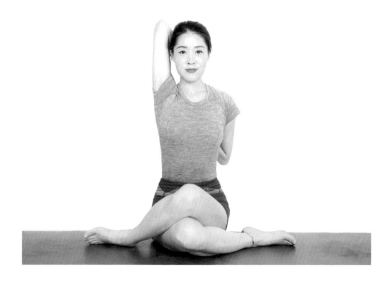

3. 跪姿体式 Kneeling poses

(15）桌子式（四角跪姿）Table pose／Goasana

跪伏在瑜伽垫上。

Kneel on the mat.

双手在双肩正下方，双膝在髋部正下方。

Put your hands directly under shoulders, and knees directly under hips.

十指张开平铺在地面上，脚背和小腿胫骨下压地面。

Spread your ten fingers onto the floor. Press the insteps and shins into the floor.

脊柱延伸，腹部微收，头在脊柱的延长线上。

Keep your spine in a long position. Belly in. Head is on the extension line of your spine.

6

顺畅地呼吸。

Breathe smoothly.

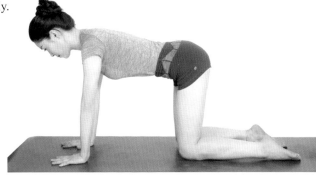

（16）猫 & 牛式 Cat & Cow pose

A　猫式　Cat pose / Bidalasana

四角跪姿开始。

Start in table pose.

呼气，尾骨慢慢向下；头部随之向下，背部拱起。

Exhale, and slowly tuck your tailbone. Lower the crown of your head, back arched.

肚脐拱向脊椎方向。

Draw your navel up to your spine.

轻轻呼吸，伸展后背紧张的肌肉

Breathe gently and extend the tight muscles of your back.

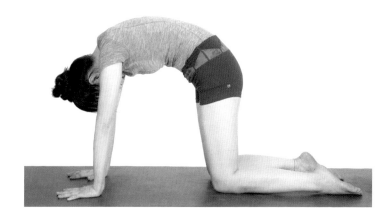

B 牛式 Cow pose / Marjaryasana

四角跪姿开始。

Start in table pose.

吸气，抬头，展开胸腔，同时坐骨向上。

Inhale, raise your head and open your chest. At the same time, lift your ischium up.

后背稍稍向下凹，眼睛向上看。

Make you back curve downward gently. Look upward.

展开肩膀，放松颈部；温和地呼吸。

Expand your shoulders. Relax your neck, and breathe gently.

6

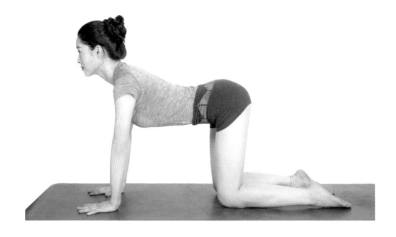

（17）交叉平衡一式 Balancing table pose/Dandayamna Bharmanasana

四角跪姿开始。

Start in table pose.

吸气，伸直左腿，脚尖点地。

Inhale, keep left leg straight, and place the toes of your left foot on the floor.

抬左腿向上与地面平行，左脚跟和脚内侧同时向后蹬。髋部保持中正。

Lift the left leg up parallel to the floor. Push your left heel and the inner side of your left foot backward. Keep your hips in the neutral position.

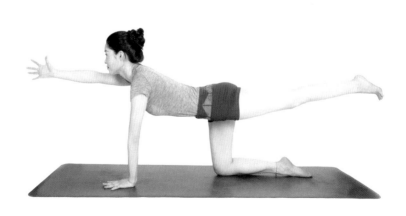

抬右手向前，右臂与地面平行。

Reach your right hand forward, right arm should be parallel to the floor.

眼睛看向右手指尖的方向，保持 3~5 次呼吸。

Gaze toward fingers of your right hand. Hold for three to five breaths.

缓慢呼气，右臂放下，膝盖收回，恢复至四角跪姿。

Slowly exhale, put the right arm down, and then lower the knee down. Back to table pose.

保持这个姿势 3~5 次呼吸，然后换另一侧练习。

Hold the pose for three to five breaths and then switch sides.

（18）骆驼式 Camel pose / Ustrasana

6

双臂侧垂，跪立在垫面上，双脚打开且与髋部同宽。

Kneel on the floor with your arms by your sides. Keep your feet hip-width apart.

小腿、脚背贴实垫面，脚尖指向正后方。

Rest your calves and insteps on the mat, with your toes pointing to the back.

双手扶髋，手肘内夹。

Place your palms on hips. Keep elbows close together.

吸气，上提胸腔。

Inhale, and lift up your chest.

呼气，大腿与垫面保持垂直，身体向后向下弯曲。

Exhale, and keep your thighs perpendicular to the floor. Throw your upper body back and down.

双手依次放在脚后跟上。

Place your hands over your heels sequentially.

展开肩膀，头自然垂落。

Expand your shoulders. Draw your head back naturally.

保持 3~5 次呼吸，双手扶髋，吸气，还原为起始姿势。

Hold for three to five breaths. Place your hands on the hips. Inhale, and return to the starting pose.

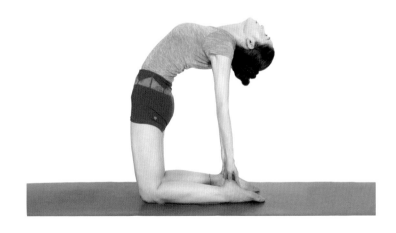

4. 俯卧体式 Lying on the stomach

（19）人面狮身式 Sphinx pose / Salamba Bhujangasana

俯卧在垫面上，双腿伸直。

Lie face down with legs straight.

双脚打开与髋同宽，脚背贴地。

Keep your feet hip-width apart. Put the insteps on the floor.

屈手肘放于双肩下方，两小臂平行放于垫面，掌心朝下。

Bend your elbows under your shoulders. Place your forearms on the mat parallel to each other, palms facing down.

大臂垂直于地面。

Upper arms are perpendicular to the floor.

6

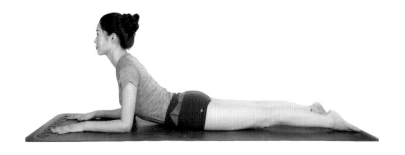

大腿肌肉收紧，脚背压地，尾骨找向脚跟。

Tighten your thigh muscles. Press your insteps into the floor. Lengthen your tailbone toward your heels.

小臂和手掌向下压地。

Press your forearms and palms into the floor.

展开胸腔和肩膀，双肩下沉，抬头向上看。

Expand your chest and shoulders. Lower your shoulders down. Lift your head up and look upward.

保持 3~5 次呼吸，呼气，放松身体。

Hold for three to five breaths, then breathe out. Relax your body.

（20）眼镜蛇式 Cobra pose / Bhujangasana

俯卧在垫面上，双腿并拢且伸直，脚背贴地。

Lie on your stomach, legs straight and together. Put the insteps on the floor.

双手放在胸腔两侧，十指打开，手肘向中线靠拢。

Place your hands by the sides of your chest. Spread your ten fingers, elbows close to the midline of your body.

大腿肌肉收紧，脚背压地，尾骨找向脚跟。

Tighten your thigh muscles. Press the insteps into the floor. Lengthen your tailbone toward your heels.

吸气，抬头，向前、向上延展脊柱，充分展开胸腔。

Inhale, head up. Extend your spine forward and upward. Expand your chest fully.

保持耻骨贴地。

Keep your pubis on the floor.

双手轻推地，手肘微屈，抬头向上看。

Push the floor gently with your hands. Bend your elbows slightly. Lift your head and look upward.

保持 3~5 次呼吸，呼气，将身体放松。

Keep three to five breaths. Exhale and relax your whole body.

还原到地面上。

Return to the floor.

6

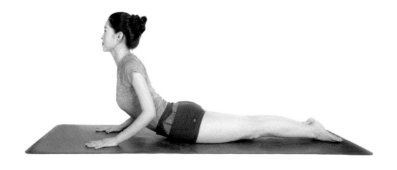

（21）蝗虫式 Locust pose / Salabhasana

A 半蝗虫式 Half locust pose / Ardha Salabhasana

俯卧在垫面上，双腿并拢且伸直，脚背贴地。

Lie face down. Keep your legs straight and together. Put the insteps on the floor.

双手掌心朝下放在身体两侧，前额点地。

Place your arms along the sides of your torso, with your palms down. Place your forehead on the floor.

吸气，大腿肌肉收紧，脚背下压，尾骨找向脚跟。

Inhale, and tighten your thigh muscles. Press the insteps into the floor. Lengthen your tailbone toward your heels.

呼气，抬右腿向上，保持右腿伸直，右侧髋部在地面上。

Exhale, and raise your right leg up. Keep the right leg straight and right hip on the floor.

保持 3~5 次呼吸，放下右腿，换至另一侧。

Hold for three to five breaths. Return the right leg to the floor. Switch sides.

B 蝗虫式 Locust pose / Salabhasana

俯卧在垫面上，双腿并拢且伸直，脚背贴地，前额点地。

Lie face down. Keep your legs straight and together. Place the insteps on the floor. Put your forehead on the floor.

双手放在身体后侧，十指交扣或掌心相对

Place your hands behind your body, with ten fingers interlocking or palms facing each other.

吸气，大腿肌肉收紧，脚背下压，尾骨找向脚跟。

Inhale, and tighten your thigh muscles. Press the insteps into the floor. Lengthen your tailbone toward your heels.

呼气，头部、胸腔、双手及双腿同时抬高并伸展，眼睛平视前方。

Exhale, lift up your head and keep your chest, hands and legs off the mat. Gaze forward.

尽量保持双脚并拢。

Try to keep your feet together.

保持 3~5 次呼吸，还原为起始姿势。

Hold for three to five breaths. Return to the starting pose.

6

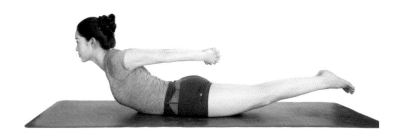

（22）弓式 Bow pose / Dhanurasana

俯卧在垫面上，双腿并拢且伸直，脚背贴地。

Lie on your stomach. Keep your legs straight and together. Place the insteps on the floor.

双手掌心朝下，放在身体的两侧，前额点地。

Place your arms along the sides of your torso, with your palms down and your forehead resting on the floor.

屈双膝，双脚脚跟尽可能地靠近臀部。

Bend your knees. Bring your heels to buttocks as close as you can.

双手向后抓住脚踝外侧，双腿分开大约一个拳头，尾骨向膝盖的方向顺延。

Reach back with your hands to hold the outer sides of your ankles. Keep your legs one-fist apart. Lengthen your tailbone down to knees.

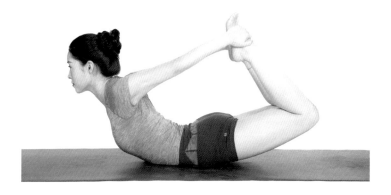

呼气，抬高大腿向上，小腿向后推，直到膝盖朝向正后方。

Exhale, and lift your thighs up. Push your lower legs backward. Knees should face directly backward.

展开胸腔和肩膀，眼睛平视前方，颈部后侧放松。

Open your chest and shoulders. Gaze forward. Relax the back of your neck.

保持 3~5 次呼吸，还原为俯卧姿势。

Hold this pose for three to five breaths. Return to the facedown position.

6

5. 仰卧体式 Lying on the back

(23) 快乐婴儿式 Happy baby pose / Ananda Balasana

仰卧在垫面上，双腿伸直，双脚打开与髋同宽。

Lie face up, with legs straight. Keep your feet hip-width apart.

双手放在身体两侧，掌心朝下。

Put your hands by your sides, palms facing down.

屈双膝，双膝打开略宽于腰部。

Bend your knees. Open them a little bit wider than your waist.

抬起双腿，膝盖慢慢靠近腹部两侧。

Lift up your legs. Draw your knees toward sides of your abdomen.

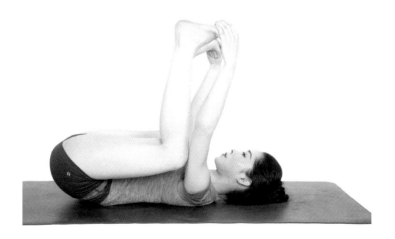

小腿垂直地面，双手握住双脚外侧。

Keep your shanks perpendicular to the floor. Grip the outsides of your feet with your hands.

呼气，双手将双腿拉向地板的方向，让体式更深入。

Exhale, and pull your legs toward the floor for a deeper stretch with your hands.

停留 3~5 次呼吸后，还原为仰卧姿势。

Hold this pose for three to five breaths. Return to the face up position.

（24）仰卧脊柱扭转 Supine spinal twist / Supta Matsyendrasana

仰卧在垫面上，双腿伸直，双脚并拢。

Lie on your back, legs straight. Keep your feet together.

双手侧平举，掌心朝下。

Extend your arms out to the sides at shoulder height, palms facing down.

6

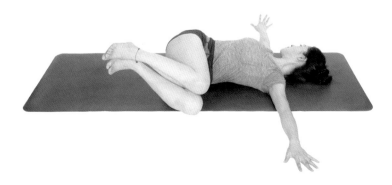

屈双膝。呼气，身体向左扭转，双膝向下靠近垫面。

Bend your knees. Exhale, and twist your body to the left. Move your knees down to the mat.

右肩压实垫面，头转向右侧。

Right shoulder is settled onto the mat. Turn your head to the right.

保持这个姿势进行 3~5 次缓慢的呼吸。

Hold this pose for three to five slow breaths.

吸气，还原为仰卧姿势；换至另一侧。

Inhale, and return to the face-up. Change to the other side.

（25）鱼式 Fish pose / Matsyasana

仰卧在垫面上，双脚并拢，双腿伸直。

Lie on your back on the mat, legs straight with feet together.

双手放在臀部两侧，掌心朝下。

Place your hands by sides of your buttocks, palms facing down.

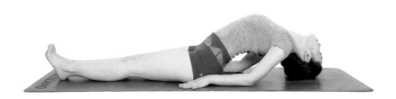

呼气，小臂及手肘推地。

Exhale, and press your forearms and elbows firmly against the floor.

胸腔上提，头部抬起，顺势滚动头部让头顶点地。

Lift your chest up, head away from the floor. Then roll your head and place the crown of your head on the floor.

向头部施加的重量要小，避免伤及颈部。

Put a minimal amount of weight on your head to avoid crunching your neck.

保持 3~5 次呼吸。

Keep three to five breaths.

呼气，身体和头回到地板上。

Exhale, then lower your torso and head to the floor.

6

（26）桥式 Bridge pose / Setu Bandha Sarvangasana

仰卧在垫面上，双腿伸直，双脚并拢。

Lie face up on the mat, with legs straight and feet together.

双手放在臀部两侧，掌心朝下。

Place your hands by the sides of buttocks, with palms facing down.

屈双膝，双脚靠近臀部。双脚分开与髋同宽，脚尖指向前方。

Bend your knees, feet close to your buttocks. Keep your feet hip-width apart, toes pointing forward.

大腿肌肉收紧，双脚内侧和外侧都踩实地面。

Tighten your thigh muscles. Press the inner and outer sides of your feet into the floor.

吸气，延展胸腔。

Inhale, and expand your chest.

呼气，抬髋部向上，双手在骨盆下方交握，胸腔靠近下巴。

Exhale，and lift your hips up. Clasp the hands below your pelvis. Bring chest up close to your chin.

大腿保持平行，小腿垂直于地面。

Keep your thighs parallel. Make your lower legs perpendicular to the floor.

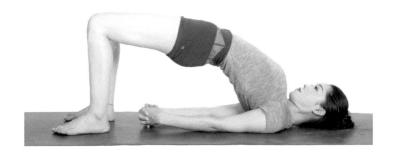

保持这个体式 3~5 次呼吸。

Stay in the pose for three to five breaths.

呼气，还原为起始姿势。

Exhale and return to the starting pose.

（27）仰卧上升腿式 Upward extended feet pose / Urdhva Prasarita Padasana

仰卧在垫面上，双脚并拢，脚趾指向天空。双手放在臀部两侧，掌心朝下。

Lie down on the back. Keep your feet together with toes toward the ceiling. Place your hands on the sides of your buttocks with palms facing down.

6

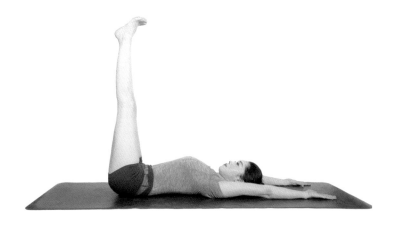

吸气，将双臂上举过头顶，手背贴地。

Inhale and raise your arms overhead. Press the back of your hand on the floor.

呼气，收紧腹部和双腿，将两腿向上抬起，与地面垂直90度，脚掌向上蹬。

Exhale, and tighten your abdomen and legs. Raise your legs off the floor to 90 degrees. Stretch your soles towards the ceiling.

尽量让腰部后侧放松，双肩下沉。

Try to relax the back of your waist. Lower your shoulders down.

呼气时，可慢慢将双腿向下移动，靠近地面。充分激活腹部核心力量。

Exhale, and move your legs down slowly. Make them close to the floor. Activate the core strength of your abdomen.

保持这个体式3~5次呼吸。

Stay in the pose for three to five breaths.

最后将双腿轻放在垫面上，还原为仰卧姿势。

Finally place your legs on the mat. Return to the face up position.

6. 支撑体式 Supporting poses

（28）下犬式 Downward-facing dog / Adho Mukha Svanasana

俯卧在地板上，双手放在胸腔两侧，十指张开。

Lie down on the stomach. Place your hands by the sides of your chest. Spread ten fingers.

双脚打开与髋同宽，脚背贴地。

Keep your feet hip-width apart. Press the insteps into the floor.

吸气，脚尖回勾。大腿肌肉收紧，手肘内夹。

Inhale，and keep your feet flexed. Tighten your thigh muscles, with elbows close to your body.

6

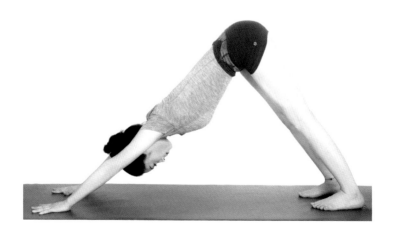

呼气，将臀部向上提到最高。

Exhale, and lift your buttocks toward the highest position.

大腿和小腿向后推，脚后跟用力向下踩，膝盖伸直。

Push your upper legs and lower legs backward. Press your heels into the ground, knees straight.

双手推地，手臂伸直。

Press your hands against the ground, arms straight.

展开腋窝，背部平展，身体呈倒"V"型。

Stretch out your armpits. Lengthen your back. Keep your body an inverted V.

保持这个体式 3~5 次呼吸，屈膝还原为俯卧姿势。

Hold the pose for three to five breathes. Bend your knees and return to the facedown position.

（29）上犬式 Upward-facing dog / Urdhva Mukha Svanasana

俯卧在垫面上，双腿伸直。双脚打开与髋同宽，脚背贴地。

Lie on the stomach. Keep your legs straight and feet hip-width apart. Place the insteps on the floor.

双手自然地放于身体两侧，前额点地。

Place your hands by the sides of your body, with your forehead resting on the floor.

将双手放在肋骨两侧，十指打开，手肘向中线靠拢。

Place your hands by the sides of your ribs. Spread ten fingers, elbows close to the midline of your body.

大腿肌肉收紧，脚背压地且向后伸展。

Tighten your thigh muscles. Press the insteps into the floor and stretch them backward.

吸气，抬头；上提胸部，双手用力推地，缓慢伸直手臂。

Inhale, head up. Lift up your chest. Press your hands into the floor to straighten your arms slowly.

腹部和双腿离开垫面，胸腔向上延展打开，双肩向后并下沉。

Lift legs and abdomen off the mat. Open your chest upward. Lower your shoulders down and backward.

保持这个体式 3~5 次呼吸，还原为起始姿势。

Hold the pose for three to five breaths. Return to the starting pose.

6

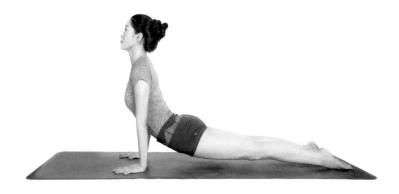

（30）平板式 Plank pose / Phalakasana

俯卧，前额点地，双脚并拢；双手放在胸腔两侧，十指张开，指尖指向正前方。

Lie on the belly. Place your forehead on the floor, feet together. Put your hands by the sides of your chest. Spread ten fingers, fingers pointing to the front.

脚尖回勾，脚后跟向后蹬，大腿肌肉收紧。

Toes flexed, press the heels backward. Tighten your thigh muscles.

双手撑地将身体向上抬，脚掌垂直于地面。

Push your hands into the floor to lift your body up. The soles are perpendicular to the floor.

保持腿、髋部和躯干在一条直线上。尾骨向脚跟延伸。同时，收紧腹部，胸腔延伸向下巴，手压实地面，双肩向后。

Keep legs, hips and torso in one straight line. Lengthen your tailbone to the heels. Tighten your belly. Lengthen your chest to the chin. Press your hands into the floor, shoulders backward.

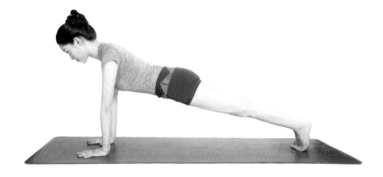

保持这个体式 3~5 次呼吸，还原为起始姿势。

Hold the pose for three to five breaths. Return to the starting pose.

（31）侧板式　Side plank pose / Vasisthasana

俯卧在垫面上，前额点地。

Lie down on your abdomen with forehead on the floor.

双手放在双肩正下方，十指张开；双脚脚尖点地，将身体向上提起至平板式。

Put hands under your shoulders. Spread ten fingers. Place your tiptoes on the floor and raise your torso to plank pose.

将重心移到右手，转身朝向左边，两脚内侧交叠，左手上举指向天花板。

Rest your weight on the right hand. Turn your torso to the left. Cross the inner sides of your feet. Raise left hand toward the ceiling.

6

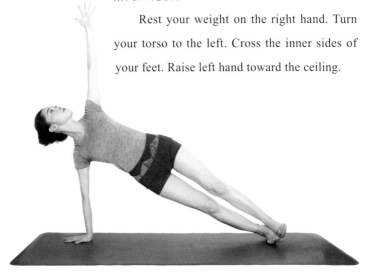

双脚内侧向前推，双腿收紧，下方腿外侧提向天花板，使身体呈一条直线。

Push the inner side of your feet forward. Tighten your legs. Lift the outer side of the lower leg up. Make your whole body in a line.

支撑手压实地面，上下手臂对抗伸展，转头看向天花板。

Press your supporting hand into the floor. Upper arm and lower arm extend together. Turn your head and gaze toward the ceiling.

呼气，落手转身向下，换至对侧练习。

Exhale, then drop your hand and turn down your body. Repeat on the other side.

第7章 瑜伽静坐调息引导口令
Chapter 7　Instruction of Yoga Meditation

静坐冥想 Meditation/Dhyana

步骤1：选择一个舒适的坐姿坐于垫子上。腰背挺直，手臂放松，双手放在膝盖上，眼睛看向正前方。翻转掌心朝上，大拇指与食指相触，形成智慧手印。闭上双眼，放松肩膀、手臂、膝盖、双脚及整个身体。

Choose a comfortable pose to sit on the mat. Keep back straight, arms relaxed. Put your hands on your knees. Look straight ahead. Turn your palms up, with the thumbs and index fingers touched into the gesture of wisdom (Jnana Mudra). Close your eyes. Relax shoulders, arms, knees, feet and your whole body.

步骤2：排除外界的一切干扰，将意识集中在呼吸上，深深地吸气，腹部慢慢地向外隆起，将新鲜空气吸入腹部；再慢慢呼气，小腹向内收，将身体的废气、浊气向外排出。保持这样的呼吸节奏，内心慢慢变得平静，抛开所有烦恼和杂念，放松身体和大脑。

Drown out any outside noise and focus on breathing. Inhale deeply and belly out, fresh air filling the abdominal cavity. Exhale the waste gas slowly, belly in. Keep this breathing rhythm. Calm inside slowly. Put aside all your worries and distractions. Ease the body and mind.

步骤 3：进入冥想练习。(5~8 分钟留白)

Get into meditation practice.(five to eight minutes)

步骤 4：再次关注呼吸，深深地吸气，慢慢地吐气，轻轻地动一动手指及脚趾，4~5 次呼吸后，慢慢睁开眼睛，放松双腿，

Focus on your breathing again. Inhale deeply and exhale slowly. Move your fingers and toes slightly. After four to five breaths, open your eyes slowly. Release your legs.

说明：静坐冥想引导词因个人需求和功能各异而通常采用不同的表达形式，以上内容仅供参考。

Note: Instruction of mediation adopt different expressions based on various personal needs and functions. The above herein is for reference only.

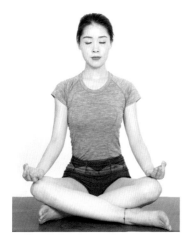
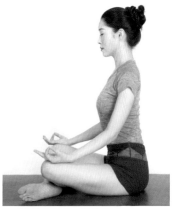

第 8 章　瑜伽休息术引导口令
Chapter 8　Instruction of Savasana in Yoga

挺尸式 Corpse / Savasana

步骤 1：仰卧在垫面上，屈双膝，抬起骨盆轻轻离开地面，双手朝向尾骨推动骨盆后侧，然后回到地板上。吸气，慢慢地压右脚跟以伸展右腿，然后再伸展左腿。放松双腿，柔软腹股沟，脚尖向外打开，柔软下背部。双手抬起头部远离颈部，放松颈部。

Lie down on the back. Bend your knees. Lift your pelvic slightly off the floor, with hands pushing the back of pelvic towards the tailbone, then return to the floor. Inhale and slowly extend the right leg by pushing through the right heel, then turn to the left leg. Release both legs. Soften the groins, and turn the feet outward. Soften the lower back. With your hands lifting the head away from the neck, release the neck.

步骤 2：你还可以用毛毯支撑头部和颈部后侧。伸展双臂朝向天花板，肩胛骨远离脊柱。再在地面上放松手臂，继而放松手背，根据舒适程度选择距身体的远近。延展锁骨，柔软舌根、鼻子和耳朵内侧，让双眼下沉。

You can also support the back of your head and neck on a blanket. Raise your arms toward the ceiling. Draw the shoulder blades away from the spine, and then release the arms on the floor. Rest the back of hands on the floor, and the distance from them to your torso should be adjusted according to comfort. Spread the collarbones. Soften the root of tongue, nose and the inner ears. Let the eyes sink to the head.

步骤 3：排除外界的一切干扰，将意识集中在呼吸上，深深地吸气，腹部慢慢向外隆起，将新鲜空气吸入腹部。再进行呼气，小腹向内收，将身体的废气、浊气向外排出。保持这样的呼吸节奏，内心慢慢变得平静，抛开所有的烦恼和杂念。放松身体和大脑。

Drown out any outside noise and focus on breathing. Inhale deeply and belly out, fresh air filling the abdominal cavity. Exhale the waste gas slowly, belly in. Keep this breathing rhythm. Calm inside slowly. Put aside all your worries and distractions. Ease the body and mind.

步骤 4：从双脚开始，依次放松身体的每一个部位。放松双脚和脚踝；放松你的双腿、膝盖、膝盖窝；感觉你大腿前侧、后侧都在不断地放松、下沉；放松你的臀部、髋部、腹股沟；感觉你的腹部在放松，后背在放松，胸腔、双肩都在放松、下沉；放松你的颈部、头部；放松你的头皮，感觉你的每一根发丝都在放松，你的身体变得很松、很松，像一根羽毛一样，轻盈地随风飘荡在空中。

Starting with your feet, ease one part of your body at a time.

Relax your feet and ankles; relax your legs, knees, and popliteal fossa. Feel the front and back of your thigh releasing down onto the floor. Relax your buttocks, hips, and groin. Your abdomen and back feel relaxed. Relax your chest and shoulders down. Feel your neck and head relaxed. Relax your scalp and feel that each strand of your hair is relaxing. Your body become light and loose like a feather, floating in the air.

步骤 5 : 进入冥想练习，想象一个美丽、平静的地方，如沙滩、草地、河边等，你享受在这美好的一切当中，变得快乐、宁静。

Get into meditation practice. Imagine a beautiful and peaceful place, such as beach, meadow, and river etc. You are enjoying yourself in this place, and become happy and peaceful.

步骤 6 : 再次关注你的呼吸，轻轻地动一动手指和脚趾，4~5 次呼吸后，呼气时，缓慢地翻转身体到右侧，继续保持 2~3 次的呼吸。睁开眼睛，再次呼气，用手压地面，抬起身体，头部最后。选择一个舒适的坐姿，双手合掌。以合十礼结束。

And focus on your breathing again. Move your fingers and toes slightly. After four to five breaths, roll gently with an exhalation onto right side. Take two to three breaths again. Open your eyes. With another exhalation, press your hand against the floor. Lift your body, and the head comes up last. Choose a comfortable sitting pose. Place your palms together. Namaste.

8

　　说明：休息术引导词因个人需求和功能各异而采用不同的表达形式和方式，以上内容仅供参考。

　　Note: Instruction of Savasana adopt different expressions based on various personal needs and functions . The above herein is for reference only.

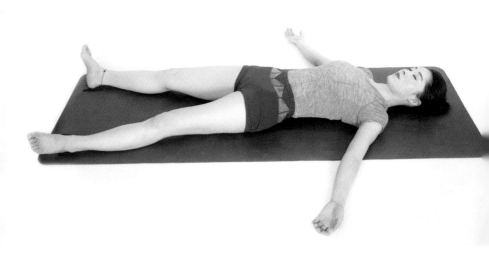

课堂主题：肩颈瑜伽

Class theme: Yoga for neck & shoulder

1. 课前沟通 Communicate with students before the class

例如：

For example :

老师：大家早上好。

Teacher: Good morning, everyone.

学生：老师好。

Student: Good morning.

老师：我是你们这节瑜伽课的老师艾薇。今天来讲解如何放松肩膀和颈部。有人患有肩膀和颈部疼痛吗？

Teacher: My name is Ivy. I am your yoga teacher in this class. Today I'm going to teach you how to relax your shoulders and neck. Does anyone feel pain in your shoulders or neck?

学生甲：我有。

Student A: Yes, me.

老师：嗯，我知道了，谁今天在生理期?

Teacher: Okay, I got it. And who are in period today?

学生乙：我。

Student B: Me.

老师：不要担心，我会多多关注你们的状况。

Teacher: Don't worry. I will pay more attention to you guys.

学生：谢谢老师。

Student: Thank you.

老师：好，那我们现在开始上课。

Teacher: OK. Let's begin our class.

说明：以上内容仅作参考。

Note: The above content is for reference only.

2. 静坐冥想 Mediation

参考第 7 章。

3. 针对肩颈疼痛的瑜伽体式序列 Yoga sequence for neck and shoulder

（1）山式 Mountain pose / Tadasana

双脚并拢。

Feet together.

脚内侧和外侧均衡地向下压。

Press the inner and outer side of your feet evenly into the floor.

大腿肌肉收紧，髌骨上提。

Tighten your thigh muscles. Pull your knee caps upward.

大腿前侧向后推，双腿垂直于地面，身体重心均匀分布在双脚上。

Turn the front of your thighs backward. Legs are perpendicular to the floor. Distribute your weight equally on the feet.

尾骨顺向地面。

Lengthen your tailbone toward the floor.

9

伸直脊柱，胸腔上提打开。

Spine straight, lift and open your chest.

双肩下沉。

Lower the shoulders down.

手臂沿身体两侧伸直向下。

Extend your arms along the sides of your body.

保持颈部、头部伸直，目视前方。

Keep your head and neck upright. Look straight ahead.

保持自然地呼吸。

Breathe normally and naturally.

（2）树式 Tree pose / Vrksasana

山式站立。

Stand in mountain pose.

左脚着地，左膝向外侧打开。

Put the toes of your left foot on the floor. Open your left knee out to the side.

抬左脚，将脚掌放在右大腿内侧。

Lift your left foot off the floor. Place the sole against the inner right thigh.

左脚脚跟靠近会阴，脚尖指向正下方。

Draw the left heel close to your perineum, toes pointing toward the floor.

右脚内侧踩实，右腿垂直于地面。

Press the inner side of right foot into the floor. Keep your right leg perpendicular to the floor.

双腿肌肉收紧，左脚与右大腿互抵用力。

Tighten muscles of your legs. Press your left foot into your right thigh, which back into your left foot with equal pressure.

髋部中正，保持身体重心的稳定。

Keep your hips in the neutral position. Keep your weight stable.

双手臂向上举过头顶，双手与肩同宽，掌心相对。

Raise your hands overhead. Open your arms shoulder-width apart, palms facing each other.

双肩放松，眼睛平视前方一个固定的点。

Shoulders relaxed, gaze at a fixed point in front of you.

保持 3~5 次呼吸，呼气，左脚落地，放下手臂。

Keep three to five breaths. Exhale, and lower your left foot to the floor. Release your arms to your sides.

换另一侧练习。

Repeat on the other side.

9

（3）鸟王（鹰）式 Eagle pose / Garudasana

山式站立，屈双膝。

Stand in mountain pose. Bend your knees.

身体重心移向右腿。

Transfer your weight to the right leg.

抬左腿向上，缠绕右大腿，左脚缠绕在右腿肚后侧。

Lift the left leg up, and twist your right left, then hook your left foot behind the lower right calf.

双手侧平举。

Reach your arms out to your sides to a T shape.

右手臂在上，左手臂在下，相互缠绕，掌心相对。

Cross your left arm under the right. Wind the right forearm around the left. Bring your palms together.

大臂平行于地面，小臂垂直于地面。

Upper arms are parallel to the floor; lower arms are perpendicular to the floor.

支撑腿的膝盖朝向脚尖，双腿收紧。

Keep your knee of the standing leg toward the tiptoes. Tighten your legs.

髋部朝前，延展背部向上。

Keep your hips forward. Stretch your back up.

保持 3~5 次呼吸。

Keep three to five breaths.

吸气，解开双腿双手。

Inhale, and unwind legs and hands.

还原为山式。换另一侧练习。

Return to mountain pose. Repeat on the other side.

（4）三角伸展式 Triangle pose / Trikonasana

山式站立，双腿分开约 1.2 米宽。

Stand in mountain pose, with your legs about 1.2 meters apart.

保持双脚外沿平行；脚趾朝前，双手侧平举。

Keep the outer edges of your feet parallel. Toes forward, reach arms out to your sides to a T shape.

转右脚 90 度，左脚微内扣。

Turn your right foot out 90 degrees to the right. Turn your left foot slightly to the right.

右脚脚跟与左脚足弓在一条直线上。

Right heel and left arch should be in a line.

右大腿肌肉收紧外旋；右膝盖与第二、三根脚趾在一条直线上。

Rotate your right thigh muscles outward. Keep your right knee in a line with the index toe and middle toe of right foot.

9

呼气，伸展躯干，身体向右、向下弯曲。

Exhale and stretch your torso. Bend your torso down to the right.

拉伸时尽量保持两侧腰等长。

Keep both sides of your torso the same stretch as possible as you can.

右手放在小腿胫骨的外侧或者瑜伽垫上。

Put your right hand on the outer side of your shin or on the mat.

左手指向天花板。

Left hand pointing toward the ceiling.

转腹部胸腔向前。

Turn your abdomen and chest forward.

转头，眼睛看向天花板的方向。

Turn your head and gaze toward the ceiling.

保持 3~5 次呼吸，吸气，蹬后腿，立直上半身。

Keep three to five breaths. Inhale, and straighten your back leg. Keep your upper body straight.

转右脚朝前；换另一侧练习。

Turn your right foot forward. Repeat on the other side.

（5）牛面式 Cow head pose/Gomukhasana

手杖式坐立，屈双膝。

Sit in staff pose and bend your knees.

将右脚从左膝下方穿过，脚背放于左臀外侧。

Cross the right foot under your left knee. Place your right instep by the outer side of your left hip.

将左脚放于右臀外侧，双膝交叠，坐骨均匀地坐实地面。

Place your left foot by the outer side of your right buttock. Cross your knees. Press your ischium into the ground evenly.

双手侧平举，左臂向上，弯曲左肘，左手掌放于上背部。

Reach out your arms to your sides to a T shape. Bring your left arm up to the sky. Bend the left elbow, and the left palm rests on the upper back.

右臂向后、向下，弯曲右肘，左右手互拉。

Bring the right arm back and down. Bend your right elbow. Your left hand and right hand should be able to hold each other.

脊柱立直，双肩展开，两手肘上下对抗，并向脊椎的中线靠拢。

Keep spine straight, stretch out your shoulders. Elbows confront each other to close the centre line of spine.

保持这个姿势 3~5 次呼吸，然后换另一侧练习。

Hold the pose for three to five breaths, and then switch sides.

9

（6）半鱼王式 Half lord of the fishes pose / Ardha Matsyendrasana

手杖式坐立在垫子上。

Sit in staff pose on the mat.

屈右膝，将右脚掌踩于左大腿外侧，膝盖指向天空；弯曲左膝，将左脚背放于右臀外侧的地面上。

Bend your right knee. Press right foot on the outer side of your left thigh. Right knee should face upward. Then bend your left knee. Place your left instep on the outer side of your right buttock.

臀部坐实在垫面上。

Sit your buttocks firmly on the mat.

吸气，手臂侧平举；呼气，身体向右侧扭转。

Inhale, and reach your arms to shoulder level. Exhale, and twist your body to the right.

右手撑在臀部后侧的地面。左手掌心朝外，手肘抵住右膝外侧。

Place your right hand behind the back of your buttocks. Palm of your left hand turn outward, with elbow against the outer side of right knee.

吸气，保持脊柱伸展；呼气，一节节从腰椎开始扭转，头转向右肩延长线。

Inhale, and stretch your spine. Exhale, twist your torso from your lumbar. Turn your head to the right and look over your shoulder.

吸气，还原，换至对侧练习。

Inhale, return to the starting position. Repeat on the other side.

（7）猫 & 牛式 Cat & Cow pose

A 猫式 Cat pose/Bidalasana

四角跪姿开始。

Start in table pose.

呼气，尾骨慢慢向下；头部随之向下，背部拱起。

Exhale, and slowly tuck your tailbone. Lower the crown of your head, back arched.

肚脐拱向脊椎方向。

Draw your navel up to your spine.

轻轻呼吸，伸展后背紧张的肌肉

Breathe gently and extend the tight muscles of your back.

B 牛式 Cow pose/Marjaryasana

四角跪姿开始。

Start in table pose.

吸气，抬头，展开胸腔，同时坐骨向上。

Inhale, raise your head and open your chest. At the same time, lift your ischium up.

9

后背稍稍向下凹，眼睛向上看。

Make you back curve downward gently. Look upward.

展开肩膀，放松颈部；温和地呼吸。

Expand your shoulders. Relax your neck, and breathe gently.

（8）下犬式 Downward-facing dog / Adho Mukha Svanasana

俯卧在地板上，双手放在胸腔两侧，十指张开。

Lie down on the stomach. Place your hands by the sides of your chest. Spread ten fingers.

双脚打开与髋同宽，脚背贴地。

Keep your feet hip-width apart. Press the insteps into the floor.

吸气，脚尖回勾。大腿肌肉收紧，手肘内夹。

Inhale, and keep your feet flexed. Tighten your thigh muscles, with elbows close to your body.

呼气，将臀部向上提到最高。

Exhale, and lift your buttocks toward the highest position.

大腿和小腿向后推，脚后跟用力向下踩，膝盖伸直。

Push your upper legs and lower legs backward. Press your heels into the ground, knees straight.

双手推地，手臂伸直。

Press your hands against the ground, arms straight.

展开腋窝，背部平展，身体呈倒"V"型。

Stretch out your armpits. Lengthen your back. Keep your body an inverted V.

保持这个体式 3~5 次呼吸，屈膝还原为俯卧姿势。

Hold the pose for three to five breathes. Bend your knees and return to the facedown position.

（9）蝗虫式　Locust pose / Salabhasana

A 半蝗虫式 Half locust pose / Ardha Salabhasana

俯卧在垫面上，双腿并拢且伸直，脚背贴地。

Lie face down. Keep your legs straight and together. Put your insteps on the floor.

双手掌心朝下放在身体两侧，前额点地。

Place your arms along the sides of your torso, with your palms down. Place your forehead on the floor.

吸气，大腿肌肉收紧，脚背下压，尾骨找向脚跟。

Inhale, and tighten your thigh muscles. Press your insteps into the floor. Lengthen your tailbone toward your heels.

呼气，抬右腿向上，保持右腿伸直，右侧髋部在地面上。

Exhale, and raise your right leg up. Keep the right leg straight and right hip on the floor.

9

保持 3~5 次呼吸，放下右腿，换至另一侧。

Hold for three to five breaths. Return the right leg to the floor.
Switch sides.

B 蝗虫式 Locust pose / Salabhasana

俯卧在垫面上，双腿并拢且伸直，脚背贴地，前额点地。

Lie face down. Keep your legs straight and together. Place the
insteps on the floor. Put your forehead on the floor.

双手放在身体后侧，十指交扣或掌心相对

Place your hands behind your body, with ten fingers interlocking
or palms facing each other.

吸气，大腿肌肉收紧，脚背下压，尾骨找向脚跟。

Inhale, and tighten your thigh muscles. Press the insteps into
the floor. Lengthen your tailbone toward your heels.

呼气，头部、胸腔、双手及双腿同时抬高并伸展，眼睛平
视前方。

Exhale, lift up your head and keep your chest, hands and legs
off the mat. Gaze forward.

尽量保持双脚并拢。

Try to keep your feet together.

保持 3~5 次呼吸，还原为起始姿势。

Hold for three to five breaths. Return to the starting pose.

（10）弓式 Bow pose / Dhanurasana

俯卧在垫面上，双腿并拢且伸直，脚背贴地。

Lie on your stomach. Keep your legs straight and together. Place the insteps on the floor.

双手掌心朝下，放在身体的两侧，前额点地。

Place your arms along the sides of your torso, with your palms down and your forehead resting on the floor.

屈双膝，双脚脚跟尽可能地靠近臀部。

Bend your knees. Bring your heels to buttocks as close as you can.

双手向后抓住脚踝外侧，双腿分开大约一个拳头，尾骨向膝盖的方向顺延。

Reach back with your hands to hold the outer sides of your ankles. Keep your legs one-fist apart. Lengthen your tailbone down to knees.

呼气，抬高大腿向上，小腿向后推，直到膝盖朝向正后方。

Exhale, and lift your thighs up. Push your lower legs backward. Knees should face directly backward.

展开胸腔和肩膀，眼睛平视前方，颈部后侧放松。

Open your chest and shoulders. Gaze forward. Relax the back of your neck.

保持 3~5 次呼吸，还原为俯卧姿势。

Hold for three to five breaths. Return to the facedown position.

9

（11）仰卧脊柱扭转 Supine spinal twist／Supta Matsyendrasana

仰卧在垫面上，双腿伸直，双脚并拢。

Lie on your back, legs straight. Keep your feet together.

双手侧平举，掌心朝下。

Extend your arms out to the sides at shoulder height, palms facing down.

屈双膝。呼气，身体向左扭转，双膝向下靠近垫面。

Bend your knees. Exhale, and twist your body to the left. Move your knees down to the mat.

右肩压实垫面，头转向右侧。

Right shoulder is settled onto the mat. Turn your head to the right.

保持这个姿势进行 3~5 次缓慢的呼吸。

Hold this pose for three to five slow breaths.

吸气，还原为仰卧姿势；换至另一侧。

Inhale, and return to the face-up position. Change to the other side.

4. 挺尸式 Corpse

参考第 8 章。

5. 课后反馈 Ask the feedback from students

例如：

For example:

老师：课程结束了，你们感觉好些吗？

Teacher: Class is over. Do you feel better now?

学生甲：我感觉好多了。

Student A: Yeah, much better now.

学生乙：但是我感到有些累。

Student B: I feel a little tried.

老师：你因为正在生理期，感到累很正常。

Teacher: That's because you are in period. Feeling a little tired is normal.

学生丙：我的腿经常会疼。下犬式这个姿势减轻了疼痛。

Student C: I feel pain in my legs. The pose Downward-facing dog has reduced the pain.

老师：嗯，我记得你是个司机，整日坐着。这个姿势会拉伸你的腿部，减轻疼痛。

Teacher: Yes. I remember you are a driver. You have to sit all day. This pose helps you stretch the leg and release the pain.

9

学生丙：好，谢谢老师，下次见。

Student C: OK. Thank you. See you next time.

老师：下次见。

Teacher: See you.

说明：以上内容仅作参考。

Note: The above is for reference only.

附录 1 词汇表
Appendix 1 Vocabulary

A

abdomen/'æbdəmən/n. 腹部；下腹；腹腔

about/ə'baʊt/prep. 关于；大约

　　　　　adj. 在附近的；四处走动的；在起作用的

　　　　　adv. 大约；周围；到处

after/'ɑːftə(r)/adv. 后来，以后

　　　　　prep. 在……之后

　　　　　conj. 在……之后

　　　　　adj. 以后的

air/eə(r)/n. 空气，大气；天空；样子；曲调

　　　　vt. 使通风，晾干；夸耀

　　　　vi. 通风

along/ə'lɒŋ/adv. 一起；向前；来到

　　　　　prep. 沿着；顺着

am/əm/abbr. 调频，调谐，调幅（amplitude modulation）

　　　　v.（用于第一人称单数现在时）是

　　　　aux.（与 v-ing 连用构成现在进行时，与 v-ed 连用构成被动语态）

and/ənd/conj. 和，与；就；而且；但是；然后

ankle / 'æŋkl / n. 踝关节，踝

anxiety / æŋ'zaɪəti / n. 焦虑；渴望；挂念；令人焦虑的事

anybody / 'enibɒdi / pron. 任何人
       n. 重要人物

apart / ə'pɑːt / adv. 相距；与众不同地；分离着
      adj. 分离的；与众不同的

arch / ɑːtʃ / n. 弓形，拱形；拱门
     adj. 主要的
     vt. 使……弯成弓形
     vi. 拱起；成为弓形

arm / ɑːm / n. 手臂；武器；袖子；装备；部门
     vi. 武装起来
     vt. 武装；备战

attitude / 'ætɪtjuːd / n. 态度；看法；意见；姿势

B

back / bæk / n. 后面；背部；靠背；足球等的后卫；书报等的末尾
     vt. 支持；后退；背书；下赌注
     vi. 后退；背靠；倒退
     adv. 以前；向后地；来回地；上溯；回来；回原处
     adj. 后面的；过去的；拖欠的

backward / 'bækwəd / adj. 向后的；反向的；发展迟缓的
       adv. 向后地；相反地

bad / bæd / adj. 坏的；严重的；劣质的；令人不适的

　　　n. 坏事；坏人

　　　adv. 很，非常；坏地；邪恶地

ball / bɔːl / n. 球；舞会

　　　vi. 成团块

　　　vt. 捏成球形

band / bænd / n. 带，环;〔物〕波段;（演奏流行音乐的）乐队；范围

　　　vi. 联合，聚集

　　　vt. 联合伙同；给……镶边；用布带绑扎；划分档次

basic / 'beɪsɪk / adj. 基本的；基础的

begin / bɪ'ɡɪn / vt. 开始；创始

　　　vi. 开始；首先

behind / bɪ'haɪnd / prep. 落后于；支持；晚于

　　　adv. 在后地；在原处

　　　n.【口】屁股

belly / 'beli / n. 腹部；胃；食欲

　　　vi. 涨满；鼓起

　　　vt. 使鼓起

belt / belt / n. 带；腰带；地带

　　　vt. 用带子系住；用皮带抽打

　　　vi. 猛击

bend / bend / vt. 使弯曲；使屈服；使致力；使朝向

　　　vi. 弯曲，转弯；屈服；倾向；专心于

　　　n. 弯曲（处）；（尤指道路或河流的）拐弯；弯道

between / bɪ'twiːn / prep. 在……之间
　　　　　　　　 adv. 在中间

big toe 大脚趾

blade / bleɪd / n. 叶片；刀片，刀锋；剑

blanket / 'blæŋkɪt / n. 毛毯，毯子；毯状物，覆盖层
　　　　　　　adj. 总括的，全体的；没有限制的
　　　　　　　vt. 覆盖，掩盖；用毯覆盖

block / blɒk / n. 块；街区；大厦；障碍物
　　　　　　vt. 阻止；阻塞；限制；封盖
　　　　　　adj. 成批的，大块的；交通堵塞的

body / 'bɒdi / n. 身体；主体；大量；团体；主要部分
　　　　　　vt. 赋以形体

bone / bəʊn / n. 骨；骨骼
　　　　　　vt. 剔去……的骨；施骨肥于

both / bəʊθ / det. 两个的；两者的
　　　　　　adv. 并；又；两者皆
　　　　　　pron. 双方都；两者都
　　　　　　conj. 既……且……

brain / breɪn / n. 头脑，智力；脑袋；聪明人
　　　　　　vt. 猛击……的头部

breath / breθ / n. 呼吸，气息；一口气，（呼吸的）一次；瞬间，瞬息；微
　　　　　　风；迹象；无声音，气音

breathe /bri:ð/ vi. 呼吸；低语；松口气；(风) 轻拂
vt. 呼吸；使喘息；流露；低声说

brow /braʊ/ n. 眉，眉毛；额；表情；山脊

buttock /'bʌtək/ n. (半边) 臀部；船尾

C

can /kæn/ vt. 将……装入密封罐中保存
aux. 能；能够；可以；可能
n. 罐头；(用金属或塑料制作的) 容器；(马口铁或其他金属制作的) 食品罐头

catch /kætʃ/ vt. 赶上；接住，抓住；感染；听见；理解
vi. 赶上；抓住
n. 捕捉；捕获物；窗钩

ceiling /'si:lɪŋ/ n. 天花板；上限

chair /tʃeə(r)/ n. 椅子；讲座；(会议的) 主席位；大学教授的职位
vt. 担任 (会议的) 主席；使……入座；使就任要职

change /tʃeɪndʒ/ vt. & vi. 改变；交换
n. 变化；找回的零钱

chapter /'tʃæptə(r)/ n. 章，回；(俱乐部、协会等的) 分会；人生或历史上的重要时期
vt. 把……分成章节

chest /tʃest/ n. 胸，胸部；衣柜；箱子；金库

chin / tʃɪn / n. 下巴；聊天；引体向上动作

　　　　　vt. 用下巴夹住；与……聊天；在单杠上做引体向上动作

　　　　　vi. 闲谈；做引体向上动作

clasp / klɑːsp / n. 扣子，钩子；握手

　　　　　vt. 紧抱；扣紧；紧紧缠绕

　　　　　vi. 扣住

class / klɑːs / n. 阶级；班级；种类；等级

　　　　　vt. 分类；把……分等级；把……归入某等级，把……看作

　　　　　（或分类、归类）；把……编入某一班级

　　　　　vi. 属于……类（或等级），被列为某类（或某级）

classroom / ˈklɑːsruːm; -rʊm / n. 教室

close / kləʊs; -z / adj. 紧密的；亲密的；亲近的

　　　　　vt. 关；结束；使靠近

　　　　　vi. 关；结束；关闭

　　　　　adv. 紧密地

　　　　　n. 结束

collarbone / ˈkɒləbəʊn / n. 锁骨

commonly / ˈkɒmənlɪ / adv. 一般地；通常地；普通地

contract / ˈkɒntrækt; kənˈtrækt / n. 合同；婚约

　　　　　vi. 收缩；感染；订约

　　　　　vt. 感染；订约；使缩短

control / kənˈtrəʊl / n. 控制；管理；抑制；操纵装置；支配权，管理权

　　　　　vt. 控制；管理；抑制

corner/'kɔːnə(r)/ n. 角落，拐角处；地区，偏僻处；困境，窘境

vi. 囤积；相交成角

vt. 垄断；迫至一隅；使陷入绝境；把……难住

adj. 位于角落的

course/kɔːs/ n. 科目，课程；过程，进程；道路；路线，航向；一道菜

vt. 追赶；跑过；奔流

vi. 指引航线；快跑

cow/kaʊ/ n. 奶牛；母牛；母兽

vt. 威胁，恐吓

cross/krɒs/ n. 交叉，十字；十字架，十字形物

vi. 交叉；杂交；横跨

vt. 杂交；渡过；使相交

adj. 乖戾的；生气的

D

day/deɪ/ n. 一天；时期；白昼

decision/dɪ'sɪʒ(ə)n/ n. 决定，决心；决议

deeply/'diːpli/ adv. 深刻地；浓浓地；在深处

desk/desk/ n. 办公桌；服务台；编辑部；〔美〕讲道台；乐谱架

door/dɔː/ n. 门；家，户；门口；通道

down / daʊn / adv. 向下，下去；在下面

　　　　　adj. 向下的

　　　　　n. 软毛，绒毛；地质；开阔的高地

　　　　　prep. 沿着……往下；在……下方；自……以来

　　　　　vt. 打倒，击败

　　　　　vi. 下降；下去；卧倒

downward / 'daʊnwəd / adj. 向下的，下降的

drop / drɒp / vt. 滴；使降低；使终止；随口漏出

　　　　vi. 下降；终止

　　　　n. 滴；落下；空投；微量；滴剂

E

each / iːtʃ / det. 每；各自的

　　　　adv. 每个；各自

　　　　pron. 每个；各自

eagle / 'iːgl / n. 鹰；鹰状标饰

ear / ɪə(r) / n. 耳朵；穗；听觉；倾听

　　　vi.〔美俚〕听见；抽穗

elastic / ɪ'læstɪk / adj. 有弹性的；灵活的；易伸缩的

　　　　　　n. 松紧带；橡皮圈

English / 'ɪŋglɪʃ / adj. 英国人的；英国的；英文的

　　　　　　n. 英语；英国人；英格兰人

equally / 'iːkwəli / adv. 同样地；相等地，平等地；公平地

everyone / 'evriwʌn / pron. 每个人；人人

example/ɪg'zɑ:mpl/n. 例子；榜样

          vt. 作为……例子；为……做出榜样

          vi. 举例；作为……的示范

exhale/eks'heɪl/vt. 呼气；发出；发散；使蒸发

         vi. 呼气；发出；发散

extend/ɪk'stend/vt. 延伸；扩大；推广；伸出；给予；使竭尽全力；
对……估价

         vi. 延伸；扩大；伸展；使疏开

eye/aɪ/n. 眼睛；视力；眼光；见解，观点

      vt. 注视，看

F

face/feɪs/n. 脸；表面；面子；外观；威信

      vi. 向；朝

      vt. 面对；面向；承认；抹盖

find/faɪnd/vt. 查找，找到；发现；认为；感到；获得

      vi. 裁决

      n. 发现

fitness/'fɪtnəs/n. 健康；适当；适合性

flat/flæt/adj. 平的；单调的；不景气的；干脆的；浅的

     adv.（尤指贴着另一表面）平直地；断然地；水平地；直接地，
完全地

     n. 平地；公寓；平面

     v. 变平；使（音调）下降

floor / flɔ:(r) / n. 地板，地面；楼层；基底；议员席
　　　　　vt. 铺地板；打倒，击倒;（被困难）难倒

fold / fəʊld / vt. 折叠；合拢；抱住；笼罩
　　　　vi. 折叠起来；彻底失败
　　　　n. 折痕；信徒；羊栏

foot / fʊt / n. 脚；英尺；步调；末尾
　　　　vt. 支付；给……换底

for / fə(r) / prep. 为，为了；因为；给；对于；至于；适合于
　　　conj. 因为

forehead / 'fɔ:hed; 'fɒrɪd / n. 额，前额

forth / fɔ:θ / adv. 向前；向外；自……以后

forward / 'fɔ:wəd / adj. 向前的；早的；迅速的
　　　　　　adv. 向前地；向将来
　　　　　　vt. 促进；转寄；运送
　　　　　　n. 前锋

front / frʌnt / n. 前面；正面；前线
　　　　vt. 面对；朝向；对付
　　　　vi. 朝向
　　　　adj. 前面的；正面的

G

gently / 'dʒentli / adv. 轻轻地；温柔地，温和地

get / get / vt. 使得；获得；受到；变成

　　　　vi. 成为；变得；到达

　　　　n. 生殖，幼兽；赢利

grasp / grɑːsp / n. 抓住；理解；控制

　　　　　vt. 抓住；领会；急切地抓

　　　　　vi. 抓

grass / grɑːs / n. 草；草地，草坪

　　　　　vt. 放牧；使……长满草；使……吃草

　　　　　vi. 长草

great / greɪt / adj. 伟大的，重大的；极好的，好的；主要的

　　　　　　n. 大师；大人物；伟人们

grip / grɪp / n. 紧握；柄；支配；握拍方式；拍柄绷带；理解

　　　　　vt. 紧握；夹紧；吸引……的兴趣或注意力

　　　　　vi. 抓住

groin / grɔɪn / n.〔解剖〕腹股沟；交叉拱

group / gruːp / n. 组；团体

　　　　　　vi. 聚合

　　　　　　vt. 把……聚集；把……分组

guide / gaɪd / n. 指南；向导；入门书

　　　　　vt. 引导；带领；操纵

　　　　　vi. 担任向导

H

happy / ˈhæpi / adj. 幸福的；高兴的；巧妙的

hardness/hɑ:dnəs/n. 坚硬；困难，艰辛，艰苦；力度；冷酷无情

head/hed/n. 头；上端；最前的部分；理解力
　　　　　　vt. 前进；用头顶；作为……的首领；站在……的前头；
　　　　　　给……加标题
　　　　　　vi. 出发；成头状物；船驶往

health/helθ/n. 健康；卫生；保健；兴旺

heart/hɑ:t/n. 心脏；感情；勇气；心形；要点
　　　　　　vt. 鼓励；铭记

heel/hi:l/n. 脚后跟；踵
　　　　　　vt. 倾侧
　　　　　　vi. 倾侧

height/haɪt/n. 高地；高度；身高；顶点

hip/hɪp/n. 臀部，髋部；蔷薇果；忧郁
　　　　　　adj. 熟悉内情的；非常时尚的

hold/həʊld/vt. 拿住，握住；持有；拥有；保存；拘留；约束，控制
　　　　　　vi. 拿住，握住；支持；有效；持续
　　　　　　n. 控制；保留

home/həʊm/n. 家，住宅；产地；家乡；避难所
　　　　　　adv. 在家，回家；深入地
　　　　　　adj. 国内的，家庭的；有效的
　　　　　　vt. 归巢，回家

hour/'aʊə(r)/n. 小时；钟头；课时；……点钟

I

important / ɪm'pɔːtnt / adj. 重要的，重大的；有地位的；有权力的

improve / ɪm'pruːv / vt. 改善，增进；提高……的价值
　　　　　　　vi. 增加；变得更好

in / ɪn / prep. 按照（表示方式）；从事于；在……之内
　　adv. 进入；当选；（服装等）时髦；在屋里
　　adj. 在里面的；时髦的
　　n. 执政者；门路；知情者

in front of 在……前面

index / 'ɪndeks / n. 指标；指数；索引；指针
　　　　　vi. 做索引
　　　　　vt. 指出；编入索引中

inhale / ɪn'heɪl / vt. 吸入；猛吃猛喝
　　　　　vi. 吸气

inside / ɪn'saɪd / n. 里面；内部；内情；内脏
　　　　　adj. 里面的；内部的；秘密的
　　　　　adv. 在里面
　　　　　prep. 少于；在……之内

instep / 'ɪnstep / n. 脚背；背部；脚背形的东西

interlock / ɪntə'lɒk / v. 互锁；连锁

inward / 'ɪnwəd / adj. 向内的；内部的；精神的；本质上的；熟悉的

ischium / 'ɪskɪəm / n.〔解剖〕坐骨

J

journey／'dʒɜːni／n. 旅行；行程
　　　　　　　vi. 旅行

K

keep／kiːp／vt. 保持；经营；遵守；饲养
　　　　　vi. 保持；继续不断
　　　　　n. 保持；生计；生活费

knee／niː／n. 膝盖，膝
　　　　vt. 用膝盖碰

kneecap／'niː kæp／n. 膝盖骨；护膝

kneel／niːl／vi. 跪下，跪

knowledge／'nɒlɪdʒ／n. 知识，学问；知道，认识；学科

L

land／lænd／n. 国土；陆地；地面
　　　　vt. 使……登陆；使……陷于；将……卸下
　　　　vi. 登陆；到达

latex／'leɪteks／n. 乳胶；乳液

learner／'lɜːnə(r)／n. 初学者，学习者

left／left／adj. 左边的；左派的；剩下的
　　　　adv. 在左面
　　　　n. 左边；左派；激进分子
　　　　v. 离开（leave 的过去式）

leg / leg / n. 腿；支柱

lie / laɪ / vi. 躺；说谎；位于；展现

　　　　vt. 谎骗

　　　　n. 谎言；位置

　　　　（过去式 lay，过去分词 lain，现在分词 lying ）

lift / lɪft / vt. 举起；提升；鼓舞；空运；抄袭

　　　　vi. 消散；升起；耸立

　　　　n. 电梯；举起；起重机；搭车

light / laɪt / n. 光，光线；灯；打火机；领悟；浅色；天窗

　　　　adj. 轻的；浅色的；明亮的；轻松的；容易的；清淡的

　　　　vi. 点着；变亮；着火

　　　　vt. 照亮；点燃；着火

　　　　adv. 轻地；清楚地；轻便地

limb / lɪm / n. 肢；臂；分支；枝干

little / 'lɪtl / adj. 小的；很少的；短暂的；小巧可爱的

　　　　adv. 不多，略微；一点儿，少量

　　　　（比较级 less，最高级 least ）

long / lɒŋ / adj. 长的；过长的；做多头的；长时间的；冗长的；长音的

　　　　vi. 渴望；热望

　　　　adv. 长期地；始终

lower / 'ləʊə(r) / vt. 减弱，减少；放下，降下；贬低

　　　　vi. 降低；减弱；跌落

　　　　adj. 下游的；下级的；下等的

M

maintain/meɪnˈteɪn/vt. 维持；继续；维修；主张；供养

master/ˈmɑːstə(r)/vt. 控制；精通；征服
　　　　　n. 硕士；主人；大师；教师
　　　　　adj. 主人的；主要的；熟练的

mat/mæt/n. 垫；垫子；衬边
　　　adj. 无光泽的

me/miː/pron. 我（宾格）

meditation/ˌmedɪˈteɪʃn/n. 冥想；沉思，深思

middle toe 中脚趾

minute/ˈmɪnɪt/n. 分，分钟；片刻，一会儿；备忘录，笔记；会议记录
　　　　vt. 将……记录下来
　　　　adj. 微小的，详细的

month/mʌnθ/n. 月，一个月的时间

morning/ˈmɔːnɪŋ/n. 早晨；黎明；初期

most/məʊst/adv. 最；非常，极其；最多；几乎
　　　　det. 大部分的，多数的；最多的
　　　　pron. 大部分，大多数

mountain/ˈmaʊntən/n. 山；山脉

mouth/maʊθ/n. 口，嘴；河口
　　　　vt. 做作地说，装腔作势地说；喃喃地说出
　　　　vi. 装腔作势地说话

move / muːv / n. 移动；步骤；迁居；策略

　　　　　vi. 移动；搬家，迁移；离开

　　　　　vt. 移动；感动

music / 'mjuːzɪk / n. 音乐，乐曲

my / maɪ / det. 我的

　　　int. 哎呀（表示惊奇等）；喔唷

myself / maɪ'self / pron. 我自己；亲自

N

neck / nek / n. 脖子；衣领；海峡

　　　　vi. 搂着脖子亲吻；变狭窄

never / 'nevə(r) / adv. 从未；决不

normally / 'nɔːməlɪ / adv. 正常地；通常地，一般地

nose / nəʊz / n. 鼻子；嗅觉；突出的部分；探问

　　　　vt. 嗅；用鼻子触

　　　　vi. 小心探索着前进；探问

noun / naʊn / n. 名词

O

of / ɒv; əv / prep. 关于；属于；……的；由……组成的

on / ɒn / adv. 向前地；作用中，行动中；继续着

　　　prep. 向，朝……；关于；在……之上；在……时候

　　　adj. 开着的；发生着的，正在进行中

open /'əʊpən/ adj. 公开的；敞开的；空旷的；坦率的；营业着的

　　　　　　　vi. 开始；展现

　　　　　　　vt. 公开；打开

　　　　　　　n. 公开；空旷；户外

out /aʊt/ adv. 出现；在外；出局；出声地；不流行地

　　　　n. 出局

　　　　prep. 向；离去

　　　　vi. 出来；暴露

　　　　vt. 使熄灭；驱逐

outer /'aʊtə(r)/ adj. 外面的，外部的；远离中心的

overhead /ˌəʊvə'hed/ adv. 在头顶上；在空中；在高处

　　　　　　　　n. 天花板；〔会计〕经常费用；间接费用；吊脚架空层

P

parallel /'pærəlel/ n. 平行线；对比

　　　　　　vt. 使……与……平行

　　　　　　adj. 平行的；类似的，相同的

peace /piːs/ n. 和平；平静；和睦；秩序

pelvis /'pelvɪs/ n. 骨盆

people /'piːpl/ n. 人；人类；民族；公民

　　　　　vt. 居住于；使住满人

perfection /pə'fekʃn/ n. 完善；完美

period /'pɪəriəd/ n. 周期，期间；时期；月经；课时；〔语法学〕句点，句号

　　　　　adj. 某一时代的

perpendicular / ˌpɜːpən'dɪkjələ(r) / adj. 垂直的，正交的；直立的；陡峭的
n. 垂线；垂直的位置

person / 'pɜːs(ə)n / n. 人；身体；人称

phrase / freɪz / n. 短语；习语；措辞；乐句
vt. 措辞；将（乐曲）分成乐句

pillow / 'pɪləʊ / n. 枕头
vt. 垫；枕于……；使……靠在
vi. 枕着头；靠在枕上

place / pleɪs / n. 地方；住所；座位
vt. 放置；任命；寄予
vi. 名列前茅；取得名次

pose / pəʊz / vt. 造成，形成；摆姿势；装模作样；提出……讨论
vi. 摆姿势；佯装；矫揉造作
n. 姿势，姿态；装模作样

practice / 'præktɪs / n. 实践；练习；惯例

practise / 'præktɪs / vi. & vt. 练习；实习；实行

press / pres / vt. 压；按；逼迫；紧抱
vi. 压；逼；重压
n. 压；按；新闻；出版社；〔印刷〕印刷机

pressure / 'preʃə(r) / n. 压力；压迫，〔物〕压强
vt. 迫使；密封；使……增压

progress / 'prəʊgres / n. 进步，发展；前进
vi. 前进，进步；进行

prop/prɒp/n. 支柱，支撑物；支持者；道具;（橄榄球中的）支柱前锋

　　　　vt. 支撑，支持；维持；使倚靠在某物上

pubis/ˈpjuːbɪs/n. 耻骨；前胸侧部

push/pʊʃ/vt. 推动，增加；对……施加压力，逼迫；按压；说服

　　　　vi. 推进；增加；努力争取

　　　　n. 推，决心；大规模攻势；矢志的追求

put/pʊt/vt. 放；表达；移动；安置；赋予

　　　　vi. 出发；击；航行；发芽

Q

quality/ˈkwɒləti/n. 质量，〔统计〕品质；特性；才能

　　　　　adj. 优质的；高品质的;〔英俚〕棒极了

R

raise/reɪz/vt. 提高；筹集；养育；升起

　　　　vi. 上升

　　　　n. 高地；上升；加薪

really/ˈriːəli/adv. 实际上，事实上；真正地，真实地;（表语气）真的吗？

relax/rɪˈlæks/vi. 放松，休息；松懈，松弛；变从容；休养

　　　　vt. 放松；使休息；使松弛；缓和；使松懈

release/rɪˈliːs/vt. 释放；发射；让与；允许发表

　　　　　n. 释放；发布；让与

remain/rɪˈmeɪn/vi. 保持；依然；留下；剩余；逗留；残存

　　　　　n. 遗迹；剩余物，残骸

represent /ˌreprɪ'zent/ vt. 代表；表现；描绘

　　　　　　　vi. 代表；提出异议

resistance /rɪ'zɪstəns/ n. 阻力；电阻；抵抗；反抗；抵抗力

return /rɪ'tɜːn/ vt. 返回；报答

　　　　vi. 返回；报答

　　　　n. 返回；归还；回球

　　　　adj. 报答的；回程的；返回的

rhythm /'rɪð(ə)m/ n. 节奏；韵律

rib /rɪb/ n. 肋骨；排骨；肋状物

　　　vt. 戏弄

right /raɪt/ adj. 正确的；直接的；右方的

　　　　vi. 复正；恢复平稳

　　　　vt. 纠正

　　　　n. 正确；右边；正义

　　　　adv. 正确地；恰当地；彻底地

roll /rəʊl/ vt. 卷；滚动，转动；辗

　　　vi. 卷；滚动；转动；起伏，摇晃

　　　n. 卷，卷形物；名单；摇晃

rotate /rəʊ'teɪt/ vi. 旋转；循环

　　　　vt. 使旋转；使转动；使轮流

　　　　adj.〔植〕辐状的

S

school /skuːl/ n. 学校；学院；学派；鱼群

　　　　vt. 教育

second /'sekənd/ n. 秒；瞬间；二等品

　　　　　　 vt. 支持

　　　　　　 adj. 第二的；次要的；附加的

　　　　　　 num. 第二

　　　　　　 adv. 第二；其次；居第二位

sequence /'si:kwəns/ n. 〔数；计〕序列；顺序；续发事件

　　　　　　　 vt. 使按顺序排列；〔生化〕确定……的顺序，确定……的化学结构序列

shank /ʃæŋk/ n. 柄；小腿；〔解剖〕胫

shoulder /'ʃəʊldə(r)/ n. 肩，肩膀；肩部

　　　　　　　　 vt. 肩负，承担

　　　　　　　　 vi. 用肩推挤，用肩顶

side /saɪd/ n. 方面；侧面；旁边

　　　　　 adj. 旁的，侧的

　　　　　 vt. 同意，支持

sit /sɪt/ vi. 坐；位于

　　　　 vt. 使就座

sleep /sli:p/ vi. 睡，睡觉

　　　　　 n. 睡眠

sole /səʊl/ n. 鞋底；脚底；基础；鳎目鱼

　　　　　 adj. 唯一的；单独的；仅有的

　　　　　 vt. 触底

spine /spaɪn/ n. 脊柱，脊椎；刺；书脊

stand / stænd / vi. 站立；位于；停滞

　　　　　　vt. 使站立；忍受；抵抗

　　　　　　n. 站立；立场；看台；停止

stomach / 'stʌmək / n. 胃；腹部；胃口

　　　　　　vt. 忍受；吃下

　　　　　　vi. 忍受

straighten / 'streɪtn / vt. 整顿；使……改正；使……挺直；使……好转

　　　　　　　　vi. 变直；好转

strap / stræp / vt. 用带捆绑；用皮条抽打；约束

　　　　　　n. 带；皮带

　　　　　　vi. 精力旺盛地工作；受束缚

strengthen / 'streŋθ(ə)n / vt. 加强；巩固

　　　　　　　　　vi. 变强；变坚挺

stretch / stretʃ / vt. 伸展，张开;（大量地）使用，消耗（金钱，时间）；使
　　　　　　　　竭尽所能；使全力以赴；

　　　　　　vi. 伸展；足够买（或支付）

　　　　　　n. 伸展，延伸

student / 'stjuːd(ə)nt / n. 学生；学者

studio / 'stjuːdiəʊ / n. 工作室;〔广播，电视〕演播室；画室；电影制片厂

style / staɪl / n. 风格；时尚；类型；字体

　　　　　vt. 设计；称呼；使合潮流

　　　　　vi. 设计式样；用刻刀作装饰画

support / sə'pɔːt / vt. 支持，支撑；支援；扶持，帮助；赡养，供养

　　　　　　n. 支持，维持；支援，供养；支持者，支撑物

switch/swɪtʃ/vt. 转换；用鞭子等抽打

vi. 转换；抽打；换防

n. 开关；转换；鞭子

T

tailbone/'teɪlbəʊn/n. 尾椎骨

ten/ten/num. 十个，十

the/ðə; ði:/art. 这；那

adv. 更加（用于比较级，最高级前）

them/ðəm/pron. 他们；它们；她们

theme/θi:m/n. 主题；主旋律；题目

adj. 以奇想主题布置的

therapy/'θerəpi/n. 治疗，疗法

there/ðeə(r); ðə/adv. 在那里；在那边；在那点上

int. 你瞧

n. 那个地方

thigh/θaɪ/n. 大腿，股

through/θru:/prep. 通过；穿过；凭借

adv. 彻底；从头至尾

adj. 直达的；过境的；完结的

tighten/'taɪtn/vt. 变紧；使变紧

vi. 绷紧；变紧

time / taɪm / n. 时间；时代；次数；节拍；倍数

　　　　　vt. 计时；测定……的时间；安排……的速度

　　　　　adj. 定时的；定期的；分期的

to / tə / adv. 向前；（门等）关上

　　　prep. 到；向；（表示时间、方向）朝……方向

today / tə'deɪ / adv. 今天；现今

　　　　　　n. 今天；现今

toe / təʊ / n. 脚趾；足尖

　　　　vt. 用脚尖走；以趾踏触

　　　　vi. 动脚尖；用足尖跳舞

　　　　（过去式 toed，过去分词 toed，现在分词 toeing）

together / tə'geðə(r) / adv. 一起，同时；相互；连续地；总共

　　　　　　　adj. 新潮的；情绪稳定的，做事有效率的

tongue / tʌŋ / n. 舌头；语言

　　　　　vt. 舔；斥责

　　　　　vi. 说话；吹管乐器

tree / triː / n. 树；木料；树状物

　　　　vt. 把……赶上树

　　　　vi. 爬上树；逃上树

triangle / 'traɪæŋgl / n. 三角（形）；三角关系；三角形之物；三人一组

twin / twɪn / vt. 使成对

　　　　n. 双胞胎中一人

　　　　adj. 双胞胎的

　　　　vi. 成对；生双胞胎

twist / twɪst / vt. 捻；拧；扭伤；编织；使苦恼

n. 扭曲；拧；扭伤

vi. 扭动；弯曲

U

under / 'ʌndə(r) / prep. 低于，少于；在……之下

adv. 在下面；在下方

adj. 下面的；从属的

up / ʌp / adv. 起来；上涨；向上

prep. 在……之上；向……的较高处

adj. 涨的；起床的；向上的

n. 上升；繁荣

upward / 'ʌpwəd / adj. 向上的；上升的

adv. 向上

use / juːz / n. 使用；用途；发挥

vt. 利用；耗费

vi. 使用，运用

usefulness / 'juːsfəlnəs / n. 有用；有效性；有益

V

vocabulary / və'kæbjələri / n. 词汇；词表；词汇量

W

waist / weɪst / n. 腰，腰部

wall / wɔːl / n. 墙壁，围墙；似墙之物

　　　　　vt. 用墙围住，围以墙

　　　　　adj. 墙壁的

water / ˈwɔːtə(r) / n. 水；海水；雨水；海域，大片的水

　　　　　　vt. 使湿；供以水；给……浇水

　　　　　　vi. 加水；流泪；流口水

wheel / wiːl / n. 车轮；方向盘；转动

　　　　　vt. 转动；使变换方向；给……装轮子

　　　　　vi. 旋转；突然转变方向；盘旋飞行

who / huː / pron. 谁；什么人

Y

year / jɪə(r); jɜː(r) / n. 年；年度；历年；年纪；一年的期间；某年级的学生

yesterday / ˈjestədeɪ; ˈjestədi / n. 昨天；往昔

　　　　　　　　adv. 昨天

you / juː / pron. 你；你们

young / jʌŋ / adj. 年轻的；初期的；没有经验的

　　　　　n. 年轻人；（动物的）崽

your / jɔː(r) / det. 你的，你们的

附录 2　瑜伽格言中译
Appendix 2　English-to-Chinese Yoga Quotes

---

*　Do your practice and all is coming.

练习吧，一切都会随之而来。

*　The hardness of a diamond is part of its usefulness, but its true value is in the light that shines through it.

– B. K. S. Iyengar

钻石本身的坚硬是它用处的一部分，但是其真正的价值在它闪耀着的光里。

——B. K. S. 艾扬格

*　Your body exists in the past and your mind exists in the future. In yoga, they come together in the present.

– B. K. S. Iyengar

你的身体成型于过去，思想开拓于未来，在瑜伽练习中，它们于现在相遇。

——B. K. S. 艾扬格

*　Yoga is a light, which once lit, will never dim. The better your practice, the brighter the flame.

– B. K. S. Iyengar

瑜伽是一盏灯，一旦被点亮，就永远不会熄灭。你练习得越好，火焰就越亮。

——B. K. S. 艾扬格

* Every morning we are born again. What we do today is what matters most.

– Gautama Buddha

每天早晨我们都经历一次重生，我们今天所要做的才是最重要的。

——释迦牟尼

* You cannot always control what goes on outside. But you can always control what goes on inside.

你总是无法控制外面的世界，但是你可以控制自己的内心。

* Five things yoga has taught me: honor your body; let go of things that no longer serve you; breathe; be present and okay with it; you can achieve more than you think.

瑜伽教给我的 5 件事：以自己身体为荣；对那些不属于自己的事放手；呼吸；关注当下；你可以得到的比你想象中的要多。

* When you are confused, it's a blessing because in confusion a concept is being broken in your mind and a new concept is being formed. This is a sign of progress.

当你感到困惑时，这其实是一种福祉。因为就是在困惑过程中，旧概念被打破，新概念得以成型。这是一种进步的迹象。

* Inhale the future, exhale the past.

吸进未来，呼出过去。

* Yoga allows you to rediscover a sense of wholeness in your life, where you do not feel like you are constantly trying to fit broken pieces together.

– B. K. S. Iyengar

瑜伽让你发现生活中的完整感，在此过程中感觉好像不断将思想中的碎片拼凑而合。

——B. K. S. 艾扬格

* You have the potential to make beautiful things. Yes, you can.

你有潜力创造出美好的事情。是的，你可以。

* Yoga is 99% practice and 1% theory.

– Sri Pattabhi Jois

瑜伽是 99% 的练习加上 1% 的理论。

——吉祥的帕塔比·乔伊斯

* The nature of yoga is to shine the light of awareness into the darkest corners of the body.

– Jason Crandell

瑜伽的本质是把意识的亮光照进身体最黑暗的角落。

——杰森·克兰德尔

* The beauty is that people often come here for the stretch, and leave with a lot more.

瑜伽之美在于人们抱着拉伸的目的来，但收获了更多离开。

* Anybody can breathe. Therefore anybody can practise yoga.

– T. K. V. Desikachar

任何人都能呼吸，因此任何人都可以练习瑜伽。

——T. K. V. 德斯卡查尔

* The quality of our breath expresses our inner feelings.

呼吸的质量展现了我们内心的情感。

* I have been a seeker and I still am, but I stopped asking the books and the stars. I stared listening to the teaching of my sole.

– Rumi

我一直都是一个追寻者，现在仍旧是，但是我不再向书本和闪耀的人物寻求，我开始听从灵魂的教诲。

——鲁米

* Yoga is not about self-improvement, it's about self-acceptance.

瑜伽不是关于提升自我，而是接受自我。

* Yesterday I was clever, so I wanted to change the world. Today I am wise, so I am changing myself.

– Rumi

昨天我自以为聪明，所以梦想改变世界。今天我变得智慧，所以我在改变自己。

——鲁米

* Yoga is like music. The rhythm of the body, the melody of the mind, and the harmony of the soul, create the symphony of life.

– B. K. S. Iyengar

瑜伽就像音乐。身体的节奏，思想的旋律，灵魂的合奏，都在创造生命和谐之音。

——B. K. S. 艾扬格

* Yoga allows you to find an inner peace that is not ruffled and riled by the endless stresses and struggle of life.

– B.K.S. Iyengar

瑜伽让你找到内心的安宁，不为生活中无尽的压力和折磨感到烦恼或被激怒。

——B. K. S. 艾扬格

* Yoga teaches us to cure what need not be endured and endure what cannot be cured.

– B.K.S. Iyengar

瑜伽教我们治愈自己不能忍受的，忍受不能被治愈的。

——B. K. S. 艾扬格

* You don't have to be great to start, but you have to start to be great.

你不必等到完美状态再去开始，但你需要开始就去追求完美。

* Yoga practice is not about perfect, it's about effort and when you bring that effort every single day, that's where transformation happens, that's how change occurs.

瑜伽练习无关乎完美，它只关乎努力；当你每天都付出努力时，也就是在见证自己的转变，领悟自己的改进。

* When you inhale, you are taking the strength from God. When you exhale, it represents the service you are giving to the world.

– B.K.S. Iyengar

当你吸气时，你从神那里汲取力量；当你呼气时，你服务于存在的世界。

——B. K. S. 艾扬格

* The pose begins when you want to leave it.

体式练习从你想要退出体式的时候正式开始。

* Life is a small gap between birth and death. So in this gap be happy and try to make others happy! Enjoy every moment of life.

人生是出生和死亡之间的一道小小的沟，所以在这道沟里，要活得快乐，努力让他人也快乐，享受生活的每一刻。

* Silence and smile are two powerful tools. Smile is the way to solve many problems and silence is the way to avoid many problems.

沉默和微笑是两个有力的工具。微笑是解决很多问题的方法；沉默是避免很多问题的方法。

* Meditation begins wisdom; lack of meditation leaves ignorance. Know well what leads you forward and what holds you back, and choose the path that leads to wisdom.

冥想始于智慧，缺乏冥想会让人无知。了解智识才会引导你前进，也会令你回望，并最终选择通往智慧之路。

* Yoga makes you stay young. It keeps the body full of vitality and immune to diseases, even at an old age.

瑜伽让你保持年轻，让身体充满活力，对疾病免疫，即使在年老的时候。

* Next time when you think of beautiful things, don't forget to count yourself it.

下次当你想到美丽的东西时，不要忘记把你自己算进去。

* How to be happy? Stop comparing yourself with others.

怎么才能快乐？停止和他人比较。

* Hold on, pain ends.

坚持，痛苦就会结束。

* Heart is a very good fertilizer; anything we plant – love, hate, fear, hope, revenge, jealousy... Surely grows and bears fruit. We have to decide what to harvest.

心灵是非常好的肥料，任何我们种植的——爱、恨、恐惧、希望、复仇、嫉妒……都会生长并结果。我们要决定的是去收获什么。

* When you're in Position of Yoga, you wait for the inner body to settle, like the water in a glass that has been placed on a table.

  当你进入一个瑜伽体位时，你的内心仿佛放在桌面的杯子里的水一样波澜不惊。

* Yoga began with the first person wanting to be healthy and happy all the time.

  –Sri Swami Satchidananda

  如果你想健康和快乐常伴，那么瑜伽是你的首选。

  ——吉祥的沙吉难陀尊者

* Yoga means addition –Addition of energy, strength, and beauty to body, mind, and soul.

  瑜伽意味着增加，增加你的能量、力量以及身体、思想、灵魂的美。

* The most important pieces of equipment you need for doing yoga are your body and your mind. That's all.

  练习瑜伽的必要设备就是你的身体和心灵，仅此而已。

* The long and uninterrupted practice of asanas done with awareness, brings success.

  有意识的、不中断的体式练习会带来成功。

* The answers you seek never come when the mind is busy, they come when the mind is still, when silence speaks loudest.

当内心忙碌的时候，你找不到一直寻找的答案；当内心安静时，它们不请自来。

* There is no competition or judgement in yoga.

在瑜伽中，不应有比较或评判。

* Inner peace begins the moment you choose not to allow another person or event to control your emotions.

内心的平静来自你不让其他人或事控制你的情感的那刻。

* Letting go is the hardest asana.

放手是最难的体式。

* Worrying does not take away tomorrow's troubles. It takes away today's peace.

担心不会带走明天的麻烦，它只会带走今天的平静。

* Meditation – Because some questions can't be answered by Google.

去冥想——因为有些问题是谷歌回答不了的。

* It's all about progress, not perfection.

只关注进步，别追求完美。

* You are stronger than you think.

你比想象中要强大。

* It never gets easier, you just get stronger.

体式练习不会越来越轻松，你只会越来越强大。

* The longest journey of any person is the journey inward.

人们经历的最长的路途是内心的旅程。

* If you learn self-control, you can master anything.

如果你可以学会自我控制，你可以掌握任何事。

* Don't let your mind play tricks on you. Over-thinking and worry is the cause of unnecessary pain. Let go and focus on what you can change.

不要让你的思想愚弄你。过度思考和担心会带来不必要的痛苦。对大多数事放手，关注你能改变的。

* You have two homes: earth and your body. Take care of them.

你有两个家：地球和身体，要照顾好它们。

* Eat more plants. Do more yoga.

吃更多植物，练更多瑜伽。

* Be the person your yoga mat thinks you are.

努力成为你的瑜伽垫想让你成为的那个人。

图书在版编目（CIP）数据

实用瑜伽英语 / 刘蕾，许蕾，王翔著 . -- 成都：
四川人民出版社，2019.5（2019.11 重印）
ISBN 978-7-220-11253-9

Ⅰ . ①实… Ⅱ . ①刘… ②许… ③王… Ⅲ . ①瑜伽—
英语 Ⅳ . ① R793.51

中国版本图书馆 CIP 数据核字 (2019) 第 031494 号

本书简体中文版由银杏树下（北京）图书有限责任公司出版。

SHIYONG YUJIA YINGYU
实用瑜伽英语

著　　者	刘　蕾　许　蕾　王　翔
选题策划	后浪出版公司
出版统筹	吴兴元
编辑统筹	王　頔
特约编辑	张冰子
责任编辑	吴焕姣　杨雨霏
装帧制造	墨白空间·张静涵
营销推广	ONEBOOK
出版发行	四川人民出版社（成都槐树街 2 号）
网　　址	http://www.scpph.com
E - mail	scrmcbs@sina.com
印　　刷	天津图文方嘉印刷有限公司
成品尺寸	143mm×210mm
印　　张	4.75
字　　数	60 千
版　　次	2019 年 5 月第 1 版
印　　次	2019 年 11 月第 2 次
书　　号	978-7-220-11253-9
定　　价	42.00 元